PARKINSON'S DISEASE DIET COOKBOOK FOR BEGINNERS

Simple, Flavorful Recipes and Expert Guidance for Better Living with Parkinson's

Kingsley Klopp

Table of Contents

Soup & Stew recipes

Important Note

Thank you for choosing the **"Parkinson's Disease Diet Cookbook for Beginners"** as part of your journey towards better health. This cookbook is designed to support your well-being with delicious, nutritious recipes tailored to those living with Parkinson's.

As you explore these recipes, please remember that individual dietary needs can vary. What works for one person may not be suitable for another. We encourage you to adjust these meals according to your specific health requirements. If you have any questions or uncertainties, don't hesitate to consult your healthcare provider or a registered dietitian. They can provide personalized advice to ensure your dietary choices align with your health goals.

Additionally, while we've provided nutritional information for guidance, these values are approximate and may vary based on the specific ingredients and brands you use. Always check labels and consider your unique dietary needs.

Furthermore, If our cookbook has brought joy to your kitchen and table, we'd be thrilled to hear about your experiences in an Amazon review. On the flip side, if you stumble upon any hiccups while exploring our recipes, don't hesitate to get in touch at kloppkingsley@gmail.com. We're here to support your cooking journey every step of the way.

We hope this cookbook becomes a valuable resource, helping you enjoy flavorful meals while supporting your health. Your journey is important to us, and we're excited to be part of it.

Wishing you health and happiness,
Kingsley Klopp

Introduction.

Imagine a world where the food you eat not only nourishes your body but also plays a pivotal role in managing the symptoms of Parkinson's disease. Welcome to the **Parkinson's Disease Diet Cookbook for Beginner**s, a transformative guide designed to support you on your journey to wellness through the power of nutrition. This book is here to help you navigate the challenges of Parkinson's with grace, offering delicious recipes that are as beneficial as they are satisfying.

Living with Parkinson's can be daunting, with its array of symptoms like tremors, rigidity, and fatigue. But what if the meals you prepare could become a crucial ally in managing these symptoms? This cookbook is your companion, filled with recipes tailored to meet the unique nutritional needs of those with Parkinson's, helping you feel your best every day.

The Power of Food in Managing Parkinson's

Did you know that what you eat can significantly impact your energy levels, mood, and overall health? The right diet can help manage symptoms, improve your mood, and even enhance your quality of life. In this cookbook, you'll discover how to harness the power of food to support your health, with an emphasis on ingredients that promote brain health, reduce inflammation, and boost energy. Picture yourself in your kitchen, surrounded by vibrant, fresh ingredients—fruits, vegetables, whole grains, and lean proteins—all waiting to be transformed into meals that not only taste great but also nourish your body and mind. Imagine cooking up a storm, knowing each dish is a step towards better health. This cookbook isn't just a collection of recipes; it's a celebration of the joy of cooking and the incredible benefits of mindful eating. Each recipe is designed with simplicity and nutrition in mind, making it easy for beginners and experienced cooks alike to whip up meals that delight the senses.

Recipes Tailored for You

What can you expect? How about a warm, comforting bowl of turmeric-infused quinoa and vegetable stew, rich in antioxidants and flavor? Or perhaps a refreshing spinach and berry smoothie that's not only packed with nutrients but also helps combat oxidative stress. These recipes aren't just about sustenance—they're about creating a positive impact on your daily life. You'll find a variety of meals that cater to different tastes and preferences, from hearty breakfasts to satisfying dinners and everything in between. The ingredients are chosen not only for their health benefits but also for their deliciousness. Cooking and eating should be joyful experiences, and this book aims to make them exactly that.

Beyond the recipes, this cookbook offers valuable insights into the connection between Parkinson's and diet. You'll learn about the importance of antioxidants, the role of fiber in digestion, and how healthy fats can support brain function. Armed with this knowledge, you'll be empowered to make informed choices about what you eat. Each section of the book provides practical tips for managing common challenges associated with Parkinson's, such as difficulty swallowing or loss of appetite. You'll also find strategies for meal planning and preparation, helping you maintain a balanced diet even on the most challenging days. Think of this cookbook as more than just a guide; it's a source of empowerment. It's about taking control of your health, embracing the healing power of food, and discovering that cooking can be a source of joy and creativity. Every recipe you try is a step towards a healthier, happier you. Let's also not forget the social aspect of cooking and eating. Sharing meals with family and friends can be a wonderful way to stay connected and uplifted. This cookbook encourages you to invite loved ones into the kitchen, turning meal preparation into a shared experience filled with laughter and love.

Are you ready to transform your approach to food and take charge of your health? With the "**Parkinson's Disease Diet Cookbook for Beginners**," you'll discover that every meal is an opportunity to nourish not just your body but also your spirit. It's time to set out on this culinary adventure, one delicious, health-boosting recipe at a time.

So, grab your apron, and let's get cooking! Embrace the journey towards wellness with open arms, and let the healing power of food support you every step of the way. This book is more than just recipes; it's a pathway to a vibrant, fulfilling life, where every bite counts towards a brighter future.

Chapter 1: Basics of Nutrition for Parkinson's Disease

Understanding Parkinson's Disease

Parkinson's Disease is a journey—one that begins subtly and gradually, often catching individuals and their loved ones by surprise. Imagine a life where the simple act of tying your shoelaces, buttoning a shirt, or even smiling becomes a Herculean task. This is the reality for millions of people living with Parkinson's Disease, a progressive neurological disorder that primarily affects movement.

What is Parkinson's Disease?

Parkinson's Disease (PD) is more than just a medical term; it's a complex condition that changes lives. It occurs when nerve cells in a part of the brain called the substantia nigra begin to deteriorate. These cells are responsible for producing dopamine, a chemical messenger that plays a crucial role in transmitting signals for smooth and coordinated muscle movements. As these cells die, dopamine levels drop, leading to the symptoms we recognize as Parkinson's.

Symptoms and Challenges

The hallmark symptoms of Parkinson's Disease include tremors, muscle rigidity, and bradykinesia, which means slowness of movement. Imagine the frustration of wanting to move your arm but feeling as if it's submerged in thick, sticky molasses. For many, tremors are the first visible sign—a rhythmic shaking that can't be controlled, often beginning in a hand or finger. Over time, these symptoms can spread, affecting both sides of the body and making everyday activities increasingly challenging.

But Parkinson's is not just about physical symptoms. It's about the emotional and psychological toll as well. Depression and anxiety are common companions on this journey, as individuals struggle to come to terms with the loss of independence and the fear of an uncertain future.

The Emotional Impact

Living with Parkinson's Disease requires immense courage and resilience. Each day brings new challenges and uncertainties. Loved ones watch as the person they know and cherish changes, sometimes slowly, sometimes rapidly. There are good days, where hope shines brightly, and there are tough days, where despair and frustration loom large.

The emotional impact extends to families and caregivers, who often bear the brunt of this relentless condition. They become unsung heroes, providing support, care, and love, often at the expense of their own well-being. The bond between patient and caregiver deepens, forged in the crucible of shared struggle and unwavering dedication.

Parkinson's Disease may alter the course of life, but it doesn't define it. There is hope in research, in new treatments, and in the unwavering human spirit. By understanding Parkinson's, we take a step towards compassion, towards better care, and towards a future where those affected by this disease can live fuller, richer lives.

Essential Nutrients for Parkinson's Patients

Managing Parkinson's Disease involves a multifaceted approach, and nutrition plays a crucial role in supporting overall health and well-being. A balanced diet can help manage symptoms, improve mobility, and enhance the quality of life for those living with Parkinson's. Listed below are the essential nutrients that can make a significant difference.

1. Antioxidants: The Body's Defense

Antioxidants are vital in combating oxidative stress, which is believed to contribute to the progression of Parkinson's Disease. These nutrients help neutralize free radicals, which can damage cells and exacerbate symptoms.

- Vitamin C: Found in citrus fruits, strawberries, bell peppers, and broccoli, Vitamin C is a powerful antioxidant that supports immune function and skin health.
- Vitamin E: Nuts, seeds, and leafy green vegetables are rich in Vitamin E, which helps protect cell membranes from oxidative damage.
- Beta-carotene: Carrots, sweet potatoes, and spinach are excellent sources of beta-carotene, which the body converts into Vitamin A, crucial for maintaining healthy vision and skin.

2. Omega-3 Fatty Acids: The Inflammation Fighters

Omega-3 fatty acids are known for their anti-inflammatory properties, which can be particularly beneficial for managing the neuroinflammation associated with Parkinson's.

- EPA and DHA: These omega-3s, found in fatty fish like salmon, mackerel, and sardines, are essential for brain health and may help slow cognitive decline.
- ALA: Plant-based sources of omega-3s, such as flaxseeds, chia seeds, and walnuts, provide ALA, which the body can partially convert to EPA and DHA.

3. Fiber: The Digestive Regulator

Constipation is a common issue for people with Parkinson's, making dietary fiber an essential component of their diet. Fiber promotes healthy digestion and regular bowel movements.

- Soluble Fiber: Found in oats, apples, and legumes, soluble fiber helps regulate blood sugar levels and lowers cholesterol.
- Insoluble Fiber: Whole grains, nuts, and vegetables are rich in insoluble fiber, which adds bulk to stool and aids in preventing constipation.

4. B Vitamins: The Energy Boosters

B vitamins are crucial for energy production and brain health. They play a significant role in maintaining nerve function, which is vital for people with Parkinson's.

- Vitamin B6: Bananas, chickpeas, and potatoes are good sources of Vitamin B6, which helps in the production of neurotransmitters.
- Folate (Vitamin B9): Leafy greens, lentils, and fortified cereals provide folate, essential for DNA synthesis and repair.
- Vitamin B12: Animal products like meat, dairy, and eggs are rich in Vitamin B12, which is important for maintaining healthy nerve cells and red blood cells.

5. Vitamin D and Calcium: The Bone Protectors

People with Parkinson's are at an increased risk of falls and fractures, making bone health a priority. Vitamin D and calcium work together to maintain strong bones.

- Vitamin D: Sunlight exposure helps the body produce Vitamin D, but it can also be found in fortified foods and fatty fish.
- Calcium: Dairy products, leafy greens, and fortified plant milks are excellent sources of calcium, essential for bone health and muscle function.

6. Protein: The Muscle Maintainer

Protein is vital for maintaining muscle mass and strength, which can help improve mobility and reduce the risk of falls.

- Lean Proteins: Poultry, fish, tofu, and legumes provide high-quality protein without the saturated fat found in some animal products.
- Timing of Protein Intake: For those taking Levodopa, the timing of protein intake is crucial. Protein can interfere with the absorption of the medication, so it's often recommended to consume protein-rich foods later in the day.

7. Hydration: The Life Sustainer

Staying hydrated is essential for everyone, but it's particularly important for people with Parkinson's to maintain cognitive function and digestive health.

- Water: Aim for at least 8 glasses of water a day, more if you are active or live in a hot climate.
- Hydrating Foods: Fruits and vegetables with high water content, like cucumbers, watermelon, and oranges, can also contribute to overall hydration.

8. Coenzyme Q10: The Cellular Energizer

Coenzyme Q10 (CoQ10) is a powerful antioxidant that helps generate energy in cells. Some studies suggest it may benefit people with Parkinson's by improving mitochondrial function.

- Sources: Organ meats, fatty fish, and whole grains are good sources of CoQ10, though supplements are also available.

Special Note

Every person with Parkinson's is unique, and dietary needs can vary. It's important to work with a healthcare provider or a registered dietitian to tailor a diet plan that meets individual nutritional requirements and addresses specific symptoms.

Foods to Avoid

Managing Parkinson's Disease involves not only incorporating essential nutrients but also being mindful of foods that can exacerbate symptoms or interact negatively with medications. Certain foods can interfere with the body's ability to absorb medication, trigger digestive issues, or worsen Parkinson's symptoms. Below is a guide on foods to avoid for those living with Parkinson's Disease.

1. High-Protein Foods

While protein is essential for muscle maintenance and overall health, it can interfere with the absorption of Levodopa, a common medication used to treat Parkinson's symptoms. Levodopa competes with dietary proteins for absorption in the small intestine, which can reduce its effectiveness.

- Red Meat: Limit intake, especially during medication times.
- Dairy Products: Milk, cheese, and yogurt should be consumed in moderation.
- Legumes and Beans: Although healthy, these can also impact medication absorption.

Recommendation: Try to consume high-protein foods during evening meals or several hours apart from medication times to minimize interaction.

2. Processed Foods

Processed foods are often high in unhealthy fats, sugars, and sodium, which can lead to weight gain, high blood pressure, and other health issues that may complicate Parkinson's management.

- Fast Foods: Burgers, fries, and other fast foods are often laden with trans fats and sodium.
- Packaged Snacks: Chips, crackers, and similar snacks contain preservatives and additives.
- Processed Meats: Sausages, hot dogs, and deli meats are high in sodium and nitrates.

Recommendation: Opt for whole, unprocessed foods that provide more nutritional value and fewer unhealthy additives.

3. Sugary Foods and Drinks

High sugar intake can lead to weight gain, increased blood sugar levels, and fluctuating energy levels, which can worsen fatigue and other symptoms associated with Parkinson's.

- Sugary Beverages: Soda, energy drinks, and sweetened teas contain high levels of sugar.
- Sweets and Desserts: Candy, pastries, and cakes are best consumed sparingly.
- Hidden Sugars: Be mindful of added sugars in seemingly healthy foods like flavored yogurts and granola bars.

Recommendation: Choose natural sweeteners like honey or fruit, and focus on foods with low added sugar content.

4. Saturated and Trans Fats

These unhealthy fats can contribute to cardiovascular disease, which is particularly concerning for individuals with Parkinson's who may already be at increased risk due to reduced physical activity.

- Fried Foods: Fried chicken, French fries, and similar foods contain high levels of unhealthy fats.
- Baked Goods: Many commercial pastries, cookies, and cakes use trans fats for longer shelf life.
- Full-Fat Dairy: High-fat cheeses, butter, and cream are sources of saturated fats.

Recommendation: Use healthier fats like olive oil, avocado, and nuts in moderation.

5. Excessive Caffeine

While moderate caffeine consumption can improve alertness, excessive intake can lead to increased anxiety, jitteriness, and disrupted sleep patterns, all of which can worsen Parkinson's symptoms.

- Coffee and Tea: Limit to 1-2 cups per day.
- Energy Drinks: Often contain high levels of caffeine and sugar.
- Certain Medications: Some over-the-counter medications for colds and headaches contain caffeine.

Recommendation: Opt for herbal teas or decaffeinated coffee to reduce caffeine intake.

6. Alcohol

Alcohol can interact with Parkinson's medications and exacerbate symptoms such as dizziness, balance issues, and cognitive impairment. It can also lead to dehydration and poor sleep quality.

- Beer, Wine, and Spirits: All forms of alcohol can pose risks, especially in large quantities.
- Mixed Drinks: Often contain high levels of sugar in addition to alcohol.

Recommendation: If consuming alcohol, do so in moderation and consult with a healthcare provider about safe limits.

7. Certain Vegetables

Some vegetables contain naturally occurring substances that can interfere with the metabolism of Parkinson's medications.

- Fava Beans: Contain levodopa, which can lead to fluctuations in medication levels.
- Fermented Foods: Sauerkraut, kimchi, and certain pickles can affect digestion and medication absorption.

Recommendation: Monitor the intake of these vegetables and consult with a healthcare provider about their impact on medication.

8. Salty Foods

Excessive salt intake can lead to high blood pressure and fluid retention, which are concerns for individuals with Parkinson's.

- Canned Soups and Vegetables: Often contain high levels of sodium.
- Salty Snacks: Pretzels, chips, and salted nuts should be eaten sparingly.
- Restaurant Meals: Frequently high in sodium, particularly fast food and takeout options.

Recommendation: Choose low-sodium or sodium-free options and use herbs and spices for flavoring.

Breakfast Recipes

1. Mixed Vegetable Juice

Ingredients:

- 2 medium carrots, peeled and chopped
- 2 celery stalks, chopped
- 1 medium cucumber, peeled and chopped
- 1 medium beet, peeled and chopped
- 1 apple, cored and chopped
- 1-inch piece of fresh ginger, peeled
- 1 lemon, peeled
- 1 cup water

Instructions:

1. Place all the ingredients in a juicer.
2. Juice until smooth.
3. Pour the juice into a glass and serve immediately.

Nutrition Info per Serving (1 glass):

- Calories: 100
- Carbohydrates: 25g
- Protein: 2g
- Fat: 0.5g
- Fiber: 5g
- Sugar: 15g

Number of Servings: 2
Cooking Time: 10 minutes

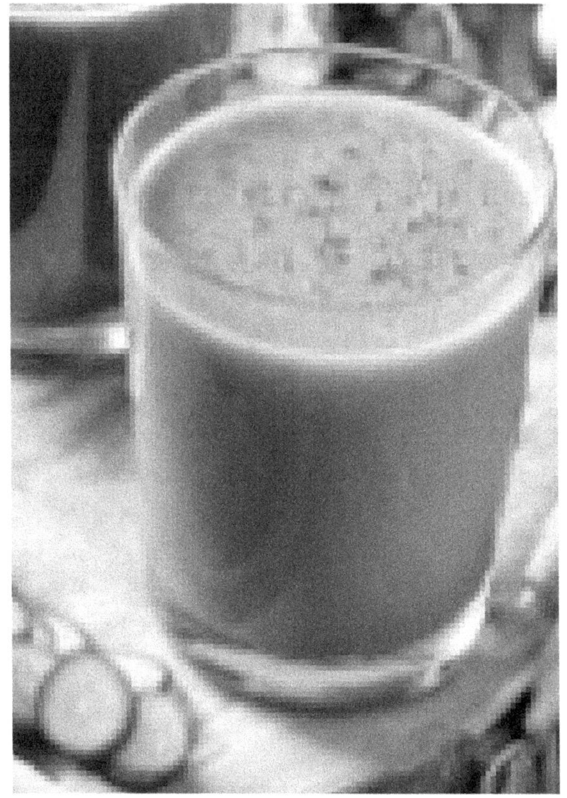

2. Tomato and Basil Bruschetta

Ingredients:

- 4 ripe tomatoes, diced
- 1 small red onion, finely chopped
- 2 cloves garlic, minced
- 10 fresh basil leaves, chopped
- 2 tablespoons extra-virgin olive oil
- 1 tablespoon balsamic vinegar
- 1 whole-grain baguette, sliced
- 1/4 teaspoon sea salt
- 1/4 teaspoon black pepper

Instructions:

1. In a bowl, combine the tomatoes, red onion, garlic, basil, olive oil, balsamic vinegar, sea salt, and black pepper. Mix well.
2. Toast the baguette slices in a preheated oven at 375°F (190°C) for 5-7 minutes, or until lightly browned.
3. Spoon the tomato mixture onto the toasted baguette slices.
4. Serve immediately.

Nutrition Info per Serving (2 slices):

- Calories: 150
- Carbohydrates: 22g
- Protein: 3g
- Fat: 7g
- Fiber: 3g
- Sugar: 4g

Number of Servings: 4
Cooking Time: 15 minutes

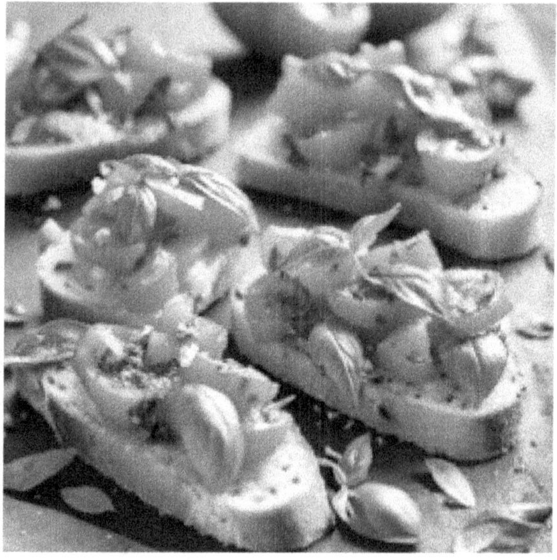

3. Savory Millet Porridge

Ingredients:

- 1 cup millet
- 3 cups vegetable broth
- 1 cup baby spinach, chopped
- 1/2 cup mushrooms, sliced
- 1 small carrot, grated
- 1 tablespoon olive oil
- 2 cloves garlic, minced
- 1 teaspoon turmeric powder
- 1/2 teaspoon cumin powder
- 1/2 teaspoon sea salt
- 1/4 teaspoon black pepper

Instructions:

1. Rinse the millet under cold water.
2. In a pot, heat the olive oil over medium heat. Add the garlic and sauté for 1 minute.
3. Add the millet, vegetable broth, turmeric powder, cumin powder, sea salt, and black pepper. Bring to a boil.
4. Reduce the heat, cover, and simmer for 20 minutes or until the millet is cooked and the liquid is absorbed.
5. Stir in the baby spinach, mushrooms, and grated carrot. Cook for an additional 5 minutes.
6. Serve warm.

Nutrition Info per Serving:

- Calories: 200
- Carbohydrates: 35g
- Protein: 5g
- Fat: 6g
- Fiber: 4g
- Sugar: 3g

Number of Servings: 4
Cooking Time: 30 minutes

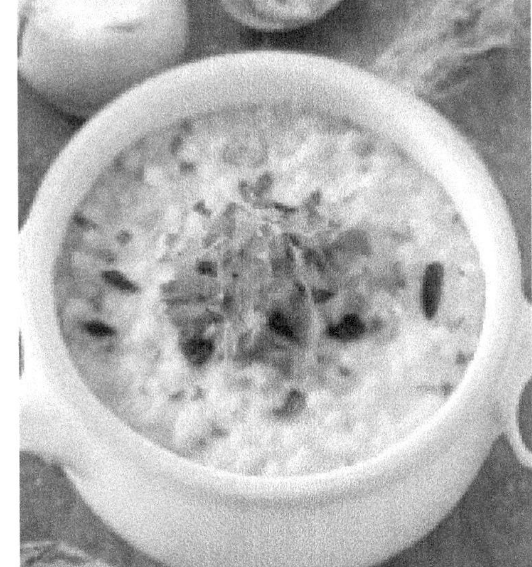

4. Papaya and Lime Salad
Ingredients:

- 1 medium papaya, peeled, seeded, and cubed
- 1 cucumber, peeled and sliced
- 1/2 red onion, thinly sliced
- 1/4 cup fresh mint leaves, chopped
- 2 tablespoons lime juice
- 1 tablespoon honey
- 1/4 teaspoon sea salt
- 1/4 teaspoon black pepper

Instructions:

1. In a large bowl, combine the papaya, cucumber, red onion, and mint leaves.
2. In a small bowl, whisk together the lime juice, honey, sea salt, and black pepper.
3. Pour the dressing over the papaya mixture and toss gently to combine.
4. Serve chilled.

Nutrition Info per Serving:

- Calories: 80
- Carbohydrates: 20g
- Protein: 1g
- Fat: 0.5g
- Fiber: 3g
- Sugar: 14g

Number of Servings: 4
Cooking Time: 15 minutes

5. Green Tea Smoothie

Ingredients:

- 1 cup unsweetened almond milk
- 1 teaspoon matcha green tea powder
- 1 frozen banana
- 1/2 cup baby spinach
- 1/2 avocado
- 1 tablespoon chia seeds
- 1 teaspoon honey (optional)

Instructions:

1. In a blender, combine almond milk, matcha green tea powder, frozen banana, baby spinach, avocado, and chia seeds.
2. Blend until smooth.
3. Taste and add honey if desired for sweetness.
4. Pour into a glass and serve immediately.

Nutrition Info per Serving (1 glass):

- Calories: 180
- Carbohydrates: 27g
- Protein: 3g
- Fat: 8g
- Fiber: 7g
- Sugar: 12g

Number of Servings: 2
Cooking Time: 10 minutes

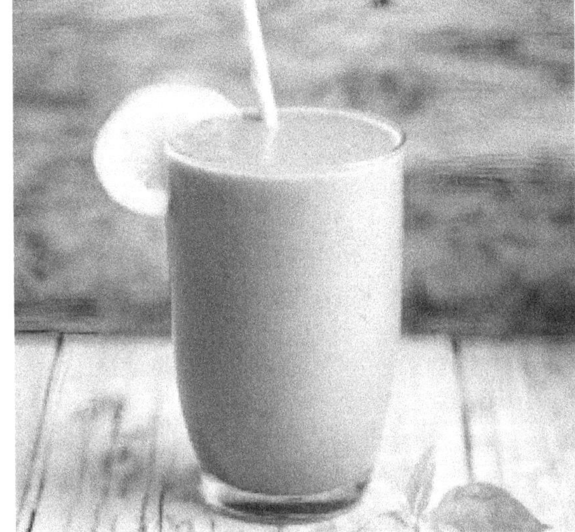

6. Raspberry Ricotta Toast
Ingredients:
- 4 slices whole-grain bread
- 1 cup ricotta cheese
- 1 cup fresh raspberries
- 1 tablespoon honey
- 1 teaspoon lemon zest

Instructions:
1. Toast the slices of whole-grain bread until golden brown.
2. Spread ricotta cheese evenly over each slice.
3. Top with fresh raspberries.
4. Drizzle honey over the raspberries and sprinkle with lemon zest.
5. Serve immediately.

Nutrition Info per Serving (1 slice):
- Calories: 180
- Carbohydrates: 22g
- Protein: 7g
- Fat: 6g
- Fiber: 4g
- Sugar: 10g

Number of Servings: 4
Cooking Time: 10 minutes

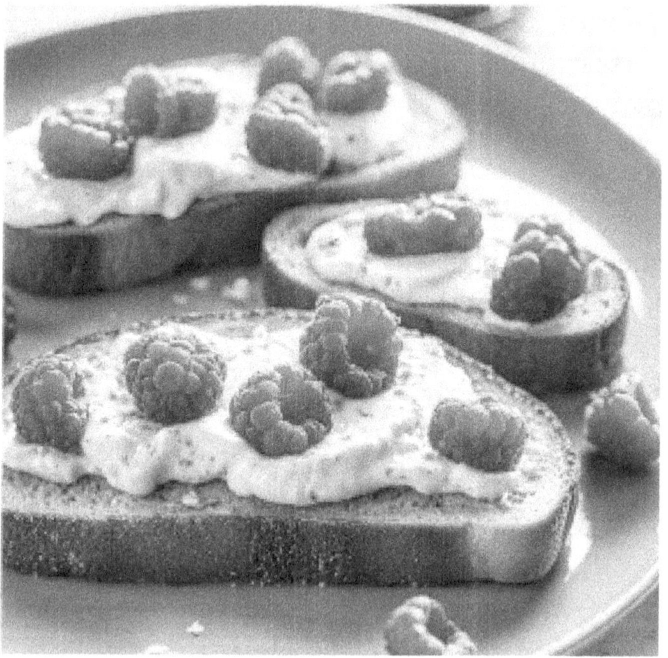

7. Almond and Date Porridge

Ingredients:

- 1 cup rolled oats
- 2 cups unsweetened almond milk
- 1/4 cup chopped dates
- 2 tablespoons almond butter
- 1 teaspoon cinnamon
- 1/4 teaspoon sea salt
- 1/4 cup chopped almonds

Instructions:

1. In a pot, combine rolled oats, unsweetened almond milk, chopped dates, almond butter, cinnamon, and sea salt.
2. Bring to a boil over medium heat, then reduce the heat and simmer for 10-15 minutes, stirring occasionally, until the oats are soft and creamy.
3. Serve warm, topped with chopped almonds.

Nutrition Info per Serving:

- Calories: 250
- Carbohydrates: 42g
- Protein: 6g
- Fat: 9g
- Fiber: 6g
- Sugar: 14g

Number of Servings: 4
Cooking Time: 20 minutes

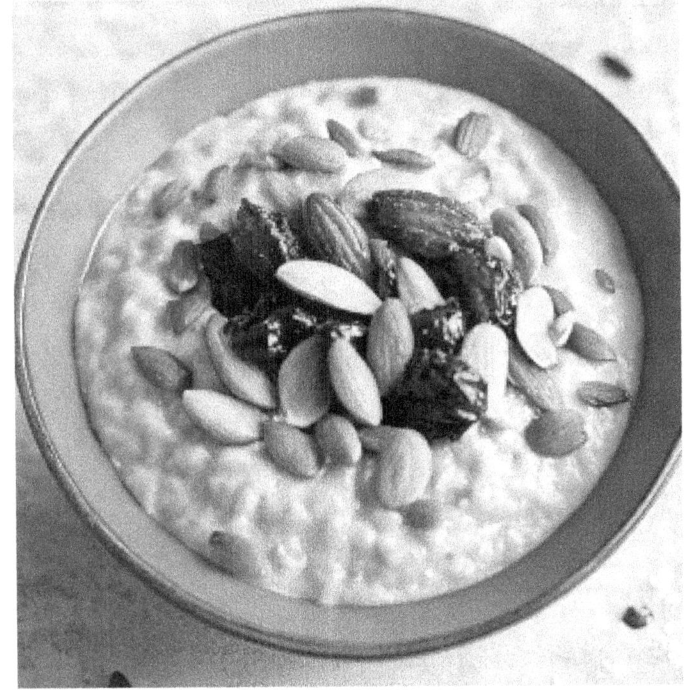

8. Overnight Chia and Oats

Ingredients:

- 1 cup rolled oats
- 2 tablespoons chia seeds
- 1 cup unsweetened almond milk
- 1/2 cup Greek yogurt
- 1 tablespoon honey
- 1/2 teaspoon vanilla extract
- 1/2 cup mixed berries (strawberries, blueberries, raspberries)

Instructions:

1. In a bowl, combine rolled oats, chia seeds, almond milk, Greek yogurt, honey, and vanilla extract. Mix well.
2. Cover and refrigerate overnight.
3. In the morning, stir the mixture and divide into bowls.
4. Top with mixed berries and serve.

Nutrition Info per Serving:

- Calories: 220
- Carbohydrates: 33g
- Protein: 8g
- Fat: 7g
- Fiber: 7g
- Sugar: 12g

Number of Servings: 2

Cooking Time: 10 minutes (plus overnight refrigeration)

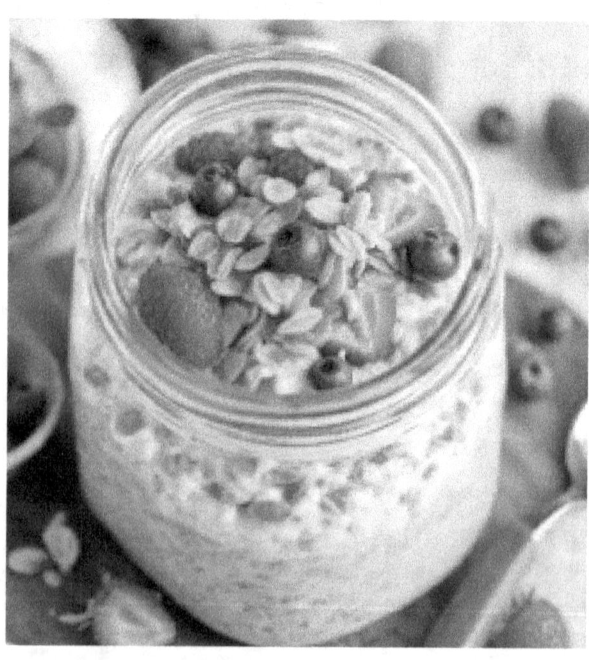

9. Salmon and Cream Cheese Bagel

Ingredients:
- 2 whole-grain bagels
- 4 ounces smoked salmon
- 4 tablespoons low-fat cream cheese
- 1 small cucumber, thinly sliced
- 1/4 red onion, thinly sliced
- 1 tablespoon capers
- 1 teaspoon fresh dill, chopped

Instructions:
1. Slice the bagels in half and toast until golden brown.
2. Spread low-fat cream cheese evenly on each half.
3. Top with smoked salmon, cucumber slices, red onion, capers, and fresh dill.
4. Serve immediately.

Nutrition Info per Serving (1 bagel):
- Calories: 300
- Carbohydrates: 45g
- Protein: 15g
- Fat: 8g
- Fiber: 5g
- Sugar: 6g

Number of Servings: 2
Cooking Time: 10 minutes

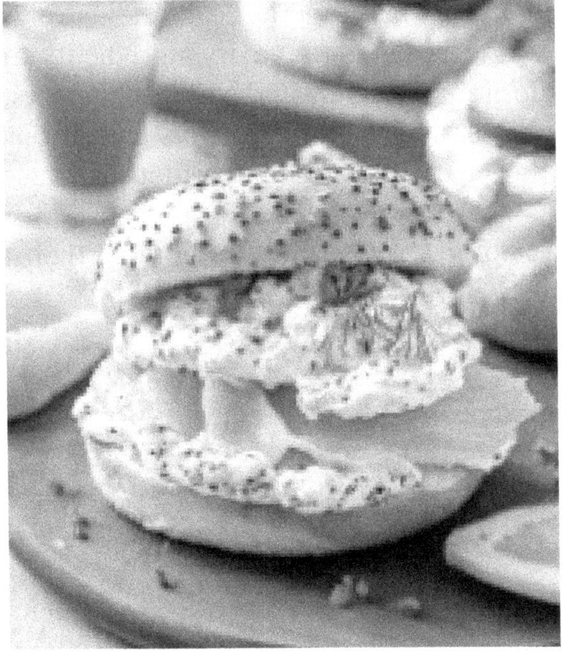

10. Zucchini Bread

Ingredients:

- 1 1/2 cups whole wheat flour
- 1/2 cup almond flour
- 1 teaspoon baking soda
- 1/2 teaspoon baking powder
- 1/2 teaspoon sea salt
- 1 teaspoon cinnamon
- 1/2 teaspoon nutmeg
- 2 eggs
- 1/3 cup honey
- 1/4 cup olive oil
- 1 teaspoon vanilla extract
- 1 1/2 cups grated zucchini
- 1/2 cup chopped walnuts (optional)

Instructions:

1. Preheat the oven to 350°F (175°C). Grease a loaf pan.
2. In a large bowl, combine whole wheat flour, almond flour, baking soda, baking powder, sea salt, cinnamon, and nutmeg.
3. In another bowl, whisk together eggs, honey, olive oil, and vanilla extract.
4. Add the wet ingredients to the dry ingredients and mix until just combined.
5. Fold in the grated zucchini and chopped walnuts, if using.
6. Pour the batter into the prepared loaf pan and smooth the top.
7. Bake for 50-60 minutes, or until a toothpick inserted into the center comes out clean.
8. Allow to cool in the pan for 10 minutes, then transfer to a wire rack to cool completely before slicing.

Nutrition Info per Serving (1 slice):

- Calories: 180
- Carbohydrates: 24g
- Protein: 4g
- Fat: 8g
- Fiber: 3g
- Sugar: 10g

Number of Servings: 10

Cooking Time: 70 minutes

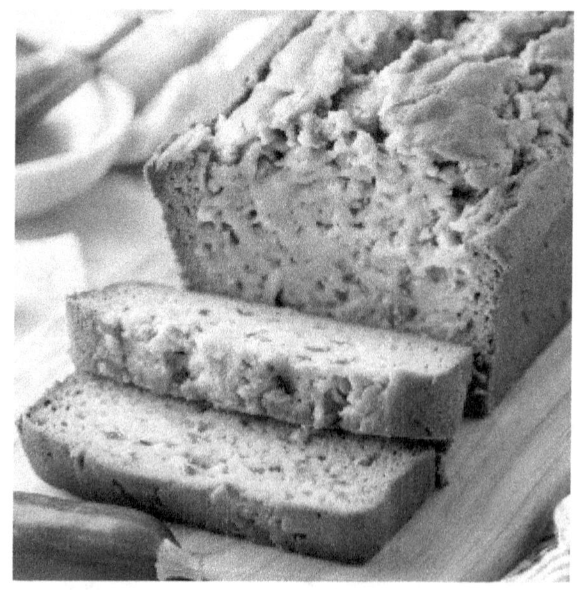

11. Beetroot and Berry Smoothie

Ingredients:

- 1 small beetroot, peeled and chopped
- 1 cup mixed berries (strawberries, blueberries, raspberries)
- 1 banana
- 1 cup unsweetened almond milk
- 1 tablespoon chia seeds
- 1 teaspoon honey (optional)

Instructions:

1. In a blender, combine beetroot, mixed berries, banana, almond milk, and chia seeds.
2. Blend until smooth.
3. Taste and add honey if desired for sweetness.
4. Pour into a glass and serve immediately.

Nutrition Info per Serving (1 glass):

- Calories: 180
- Carbohydrates: 38g
- Protein: 3g
- Fat: 4g
- Fiber: 8g
- Sugar: 24g

Number of Servings: 2

Cooking Time: 10 minutes

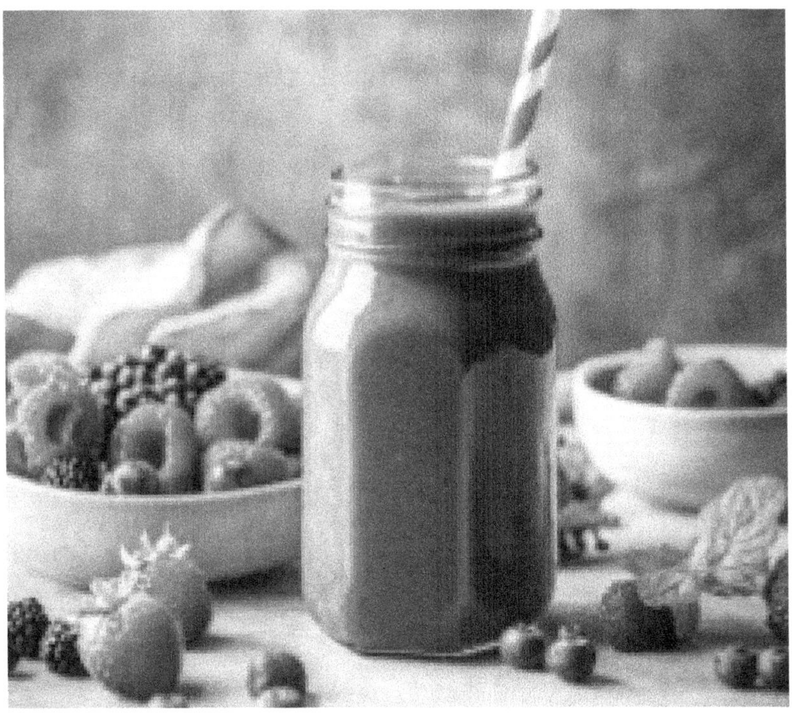

12. Blueberry and Lemon Muffins

Ingredients:

- 1 1/2 cups whole wheat flour
- 1/2 cup almond flour
- 1/2 cup rolled oats
- 1 teaspoon baking soda
- 1/2 teaspoon baking powder
- 1/4 teaspoon sea salt
- 1 teaspoon cinnamon
- 2 eggs
- 1/2 cup honey
- 1/2 cup unsweetened applesauce
- 1/4 cup olive oil
- 1 teaspoon vanilla extract
- Zest of 1 lemon
- 1 cup fresh blueberries

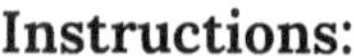

Instructions:

1. Preheat the oven to 350°F (175°C). Line a muffin tin with paper liners.
2. In a large bowl, combine whole wheat flour, almond flour, rolled oats, baking soda, baking powder, sea salt, and cinnamon.
3. In another bowl, whisk together eggs, honey, applesauce, olive oil, vanilla extract, and lemon zest.
4. Add the wet ingredients to the dry ingredients and mix until just combined.
5. Fold in the blueberries.
6. Divide the batter evenly among the muffin cups.
7. Bake for 20-25 minutes, or until a toothpick inserted into the center comes out clean.
8. Allow to cool in the tin for 10 minutes, then transfer to a wire rack to cool completely.

Nutrition Info per Serving (1 muffin):

- Calories: 180
- Carbohydrates: 28g
- Protein: 4g
- Fat: 6g
- Fiber: 4g
- Sugar: 14g

Number of Servings: 12 muffins
Cooking Time: 35 minutes

13. Bircher Muesli

Ingredients:

- 1 cup rolled oats
- 1/2 cup unsweetened almond milk
- 1/2 cup Greek yogurt
- 1 apple, grated
- 1/4 cup raisins
- 1/4 cup chopped almonds
- 1 tablespoon chia seeds
- 1 tablespoon honey
- 1/2 teaspoon cinnamon

Instructions:

1. In a large bowl, combine rolled oats, almond milk, Greek yogurt, grated apple, raisins, chopped almonds, chia seeds, honey, and cinnamon.
2. Mix well to combine.
3. Cover and refrigerate overnight.
4. In the morning, stir the mixture and divide into bowls.
5. Serve chilled.

Nutrition Info per Serving:

- Calories: 250
- Carbohydrates: 40g
- Protein: 8g
- Fat: 8g
- Fiber: 6g
- Sugar: 18g

Number of Servings: 4

Cooking Time: 10 minutes (plus overnight refrigeration

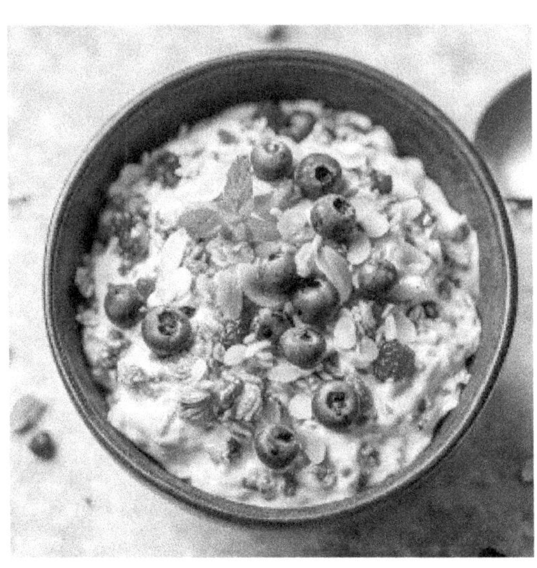

14. Pear and Walnut Baked Oatmeal

Ingredients:

- 2 cups rolled oats
- 1 teaspoon baking powder
- 1/2 teaspoon cinnamon
- 1/4 teaspoon nutmeg
- 1/4 teaspoon sea salt
- 2 cups unsweetened almond milk
- 1/4 cup honey
- 2 tablespoons olive oil
- 1 teaspoon vanilla extract
- 2 pears, peeled and diced
- 1/2 cup chopped walnuts

Instructions:

1. Preheat the oven to 350°F (175°C). Grease a baking dish.
2. In a large bowl, combine rolled oats, baking powder, cinnamon, nutmeg, and sea salt.
3. In another bowl, whisk together almond milk, honey, olive oil, and vanilla extract.
4. Add the wet ingredients to the dry ingredients and mix until well combined.
5. Fold in the diced pears and chopped walnuts.
6. Pour the mixture into the prepared baking dish and smooth the top.
7. Bake for 35-40 minutes, or until the top is golden brown and the oatmeal is set.
8. Allow to cool slightly before serving.

Nutrition Info per Serving:

- Calories: 220
- Carbohydrates: 34g
- Protein: 5g
- Fat: 8g
- Fiber: 5g
- Sugar: 14g

Number of Servings: 6

Cooking Time: 45 minutes

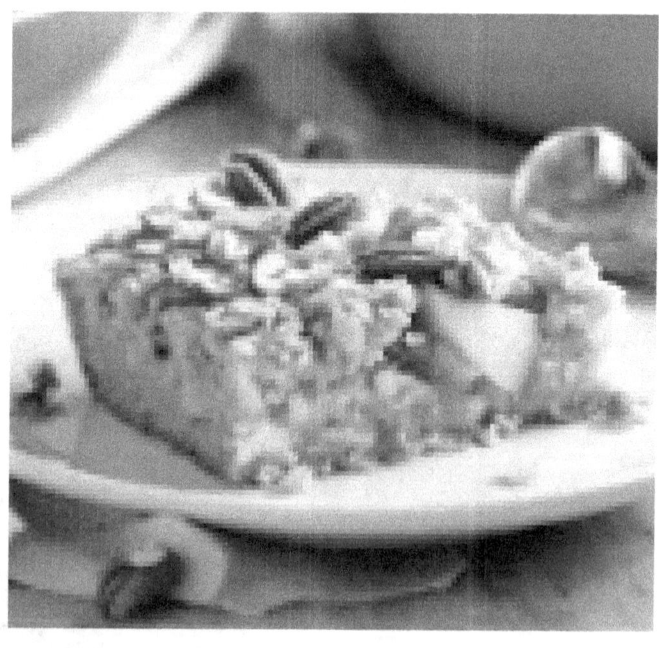

15. Mushroom and Zucchini Saute

Ingredients:

- 1 tablespoon olive oil
- 2 cups sliced mushrooms
- 1 large zucchini, sliced
- 1 small onion, thinly sliced
- 2 cloves garlic, minced
- 1/2 teaspoon dried thyme
- 1/4 teaspoon sea salt
- 1/4 teaspoon black pepper
- 1/4 cup chopped fresh parsley

Instructions:

1. In a large skillet, heat the olive oil over medium heat.
2. Add the sliced mushrooms, zucchini, and onion. Sauté for 5-7 minutes, or until the vegetables are tender.
3. Add the garlic, dried thyme, sea salt, and black pepper. Cook for an additional 2-3 minutes, stirring frequently.
4. Remove from heat and stir in the chopped fresh parsley.
5. Serve warm.

Nutrition Info per Serving:

- Calories: 100
- Carbohydrates: 8g
- Protein: 3g
- Fat: 7g
- Fiber: 2g
- Sugar: 4g

Number of Servings: 4
Cooking Time: 15 minutes

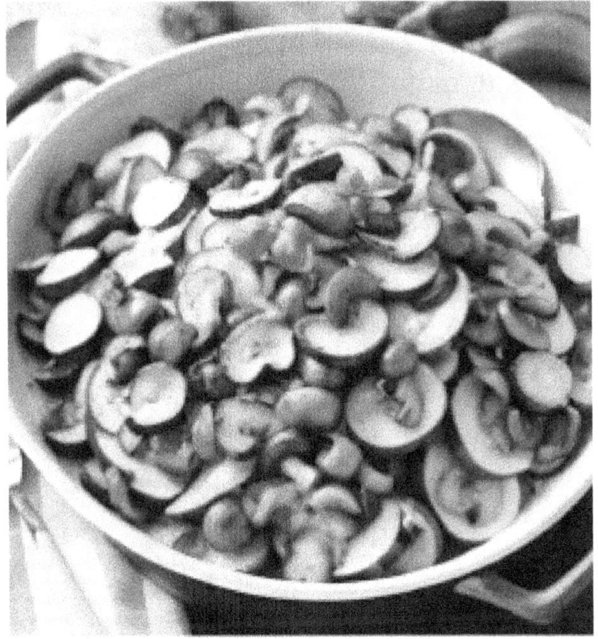

16. Pumpkin Smoothie

Ingredients:

- 1 cup unsweetened almond milk
- 1/2 cup pumpkin puree
- 1 banana
- 1/2 teaspoon cinnamon
- 1/4 teaspoon nutmeg
- 1 tablespoon chia seeds
- 1 teaspoon honey (optional)

Instructions:

1. In a blender, combine almond milk, pumpkin puree, banana, cinnamon, nutmeg, and chia seeds.
2. Blend until smooth.
3. Taste and add honey if desired for sweetness.
4. Pour into a glass and serve immediately.

Nutrition Info per Serving (1 glass):

- Calories: 150
- Carbohydrates: 32g
- Protein: 3g
- Fat: 3g
- Fiber: 6g
- Sugar: 16g

Number of Servings: 2

Cooking Time: 10 minutes

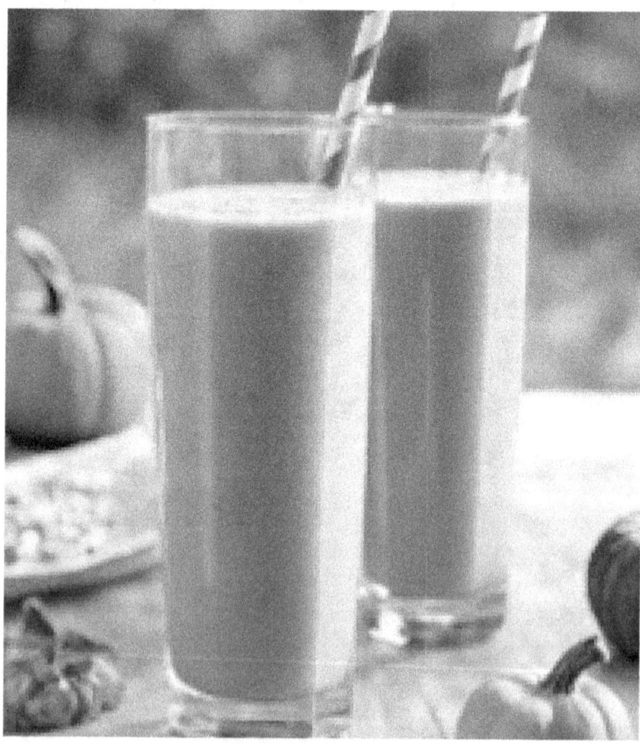

17. Apple-Cinnamon Steel-Cut Oats

Ingredients:

- 1 cup steel-cut oats
- 4 cups water
- 1 apple, peeled and diced
- 1 teaspoon cinnamon
- 1/4 teaspoon nutmeg
- 1/4 cup raisins
- 1 tablespoon honey
- 1/4 cup chopped walnuts (optional)

Instructions:

1. In a pot, bring the water to a boil. Add the steel-cut oats and reduce the heat to a simmer.
2. Cook for 20-25 minutes, stirring occasionally.
3. Add the diced apple, cinnamon, nutmeg, raisins, and honey. Cook for an additional 10 minutes, stirring frequently, until the oats are tender.
4. Serve warm, topped with chopped walnuts if desired.

Nutrition Info per Serving:

- Calories: 250
- Carbohydrates: 48g
- Protein: 6g
- Fat: 5g
- Fiber: 7g
- Sugar: 18g

Number of Servings: 4
Cooking Time: 35 minutes

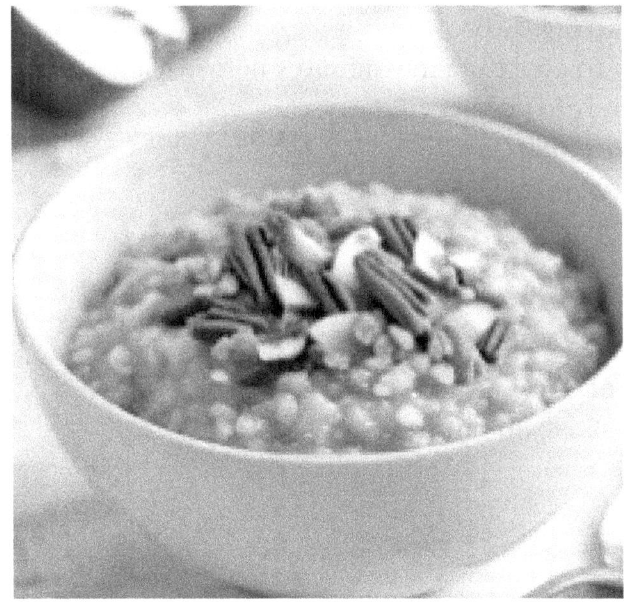

18. Kale and Sweet Onion Frittata
Ingredients:
- 1 tablespoon olive oil
- 1 small sweet onion, thinly sliced
- 2 cups chopped kale
- 6 large eggs
- 1/4 cup unsweetened almond milk
- 1/4 teaspoon sea salt
- 1/4 teaspoon black pepper
- 1/4 cup grated Parmesan cheese

Instructions:
1. Preheat the oven to 375°F (190°C).
2. In an oven-safe skillet, heat the olive oil over medium heat. Add the sweet onion and sauté for 5 minutes, until softened.
3. Add the chopped kale and cook for another 3-4 minutes, until wilted.
4. In a bowl, whisk together the eggs, almond milk, sea salt, and black pepper.
5. Pour the egg mixture over the vegetables in the skillet and sprinkle with grated Parmesan cheese.
6. Cook on the stovetop for 2-3 minutes, until the edges begin to set.
7. Transfer the skillet to the oven and bake for 15-20 minutes, until the frittata is set and lightly browned.
8. Allow to cool for a few minutes before slicing and serving.

Nutrition Info per Serving:
- Calories: 180
- Carbohydrates: 6g
- Protein: 12g
- Fat: 12g
- Fiber: 2g
- Sugar: 2g

Number of Servings: 4
Cooking Time: 30 minutes

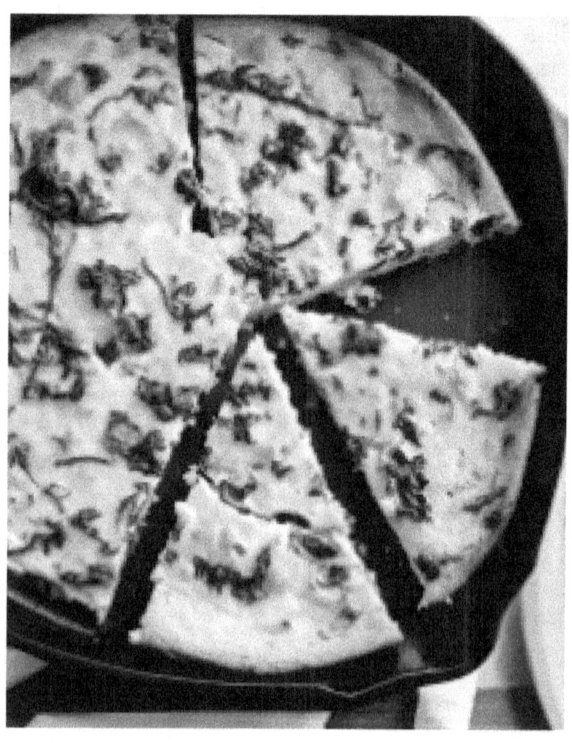

19. Rice Cake with Almond Butter

Ingredients:

- 4 whole-grain rice cakes
- 1/4 cup almond butter
- 1 banana, sliced
- 1 tablespoon chia seeds
- 1 teaspoon honey

Instructions:

1. Spread a tablespoon of almond butter on each rice cake.
2. Top with banana slices.
3. Sprinkle with chia seeds.
4. Drizzle with honey.
5. Serve immediately.

Nutrition Info per Serving (1 rice cake):

- Calories: 160
- Carbohydrates: 20g
- Protein: 4g
- Fat: 8g
- Fiber: 4g
- Sugar: 8g

Number of Servings: 4
Cooking Time: 5 minutes

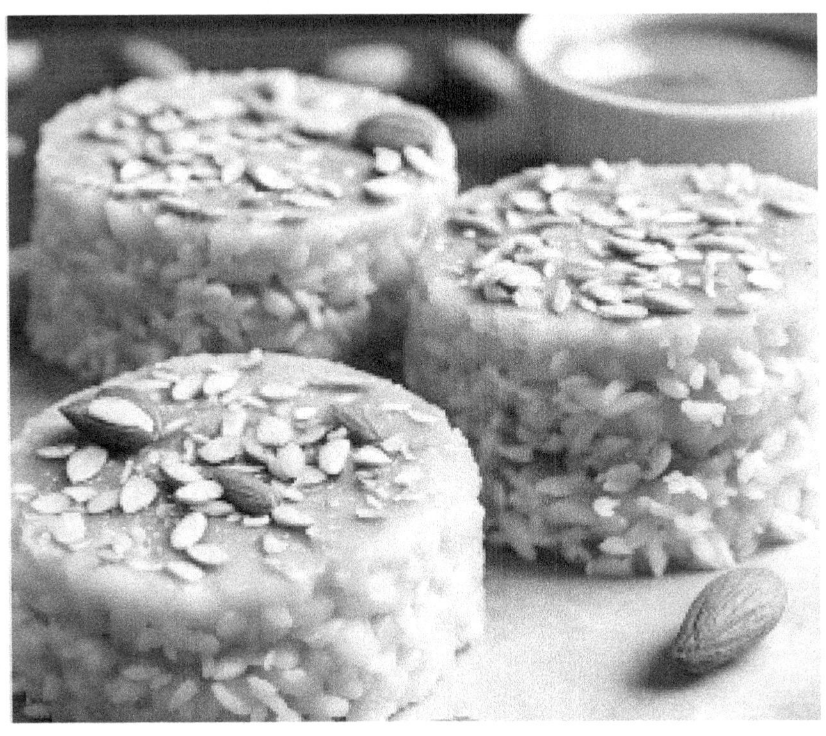

20. Buckwheat Pancakes

Ingredients:

- 1 cup buckwheat flour
- 1 teaspoon baking powder
- 1/2 teaspoon baking soda
- 1/4 teaspoon sea salt
- 1 tablespoon honey
- 1 large egg
- 1 cup unsweetened almond milk
- 1 tablespoon olive oil
- 1 teaspoon vanilla extract
- Fresh berries for topping (optional)
- Maple syrup for serving (optional)

Instructions:

1. In a large bowl, combine buckwheat flour, baking powder, baking soda, and sea salt.
2. In another bowl, whisk together honey, egg, almond milk, olive oil, and vanilla extract.
3. Pour the wet ingredients into the dry ingredients and mix until just combined.
4. Heat a non-stick skillet or griddle over medium heat and lightly grease with a bit of olive oil.
5. Pour 1/4 cup of batter onto the skillet for each pancake. Cook until bubbles form on the surface and the edges look set, about 2-3 minutes. Flip and cook for another 1-2 minutes, until golden brown.
6. Serve warm, topped with fresh berries and maple syrup if desired.

Nutrition Info per Serving (2 pancakes):

- Calories: 150
- Carbohydrates: 24g
- Protein: 4g
- Fat: 4g
- Fiber: 3g
- Sugar: 6g

Number of Servings: 4

Cooking Time: 20 minutes

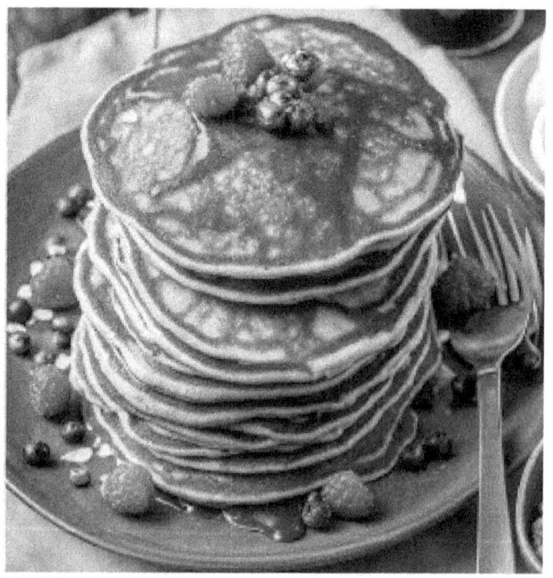

21. Muesli and Skim Milk

Ingredients:

- 1 cup rolled oats
- 1/2 cup chopped nuts (e.g., almonds, walnuts)
- 1/2 cup dried fruit (e.g., raisins, dried cranberries)
- 1/4 cup sunflower seeds
- 1 teaspoon cinnamon
- 2 cups skim milk

Instructions:

1. In a large bowl, combine rolled oats, chopped nuts, dried fruit, sunflower seeds, and cinnamon.
2. Divide the mixture into four servings.
3. Pour 1/2 cup of skim milk over each serving.
4. Let it sit for a few minutes to soften, or refrigerate overnight for a softer texture.
5. Serve chilled.

Nutrition Info per Serving:

- Calories: 300
- Carbohydrates: 45g
- Protein: 10g
- Fat: 10g
- Fiber: 6g
- Sugar: 15g

Number of Servings: 4
Cooking Time: 5 minutes (plus optional overnight refrigeration)

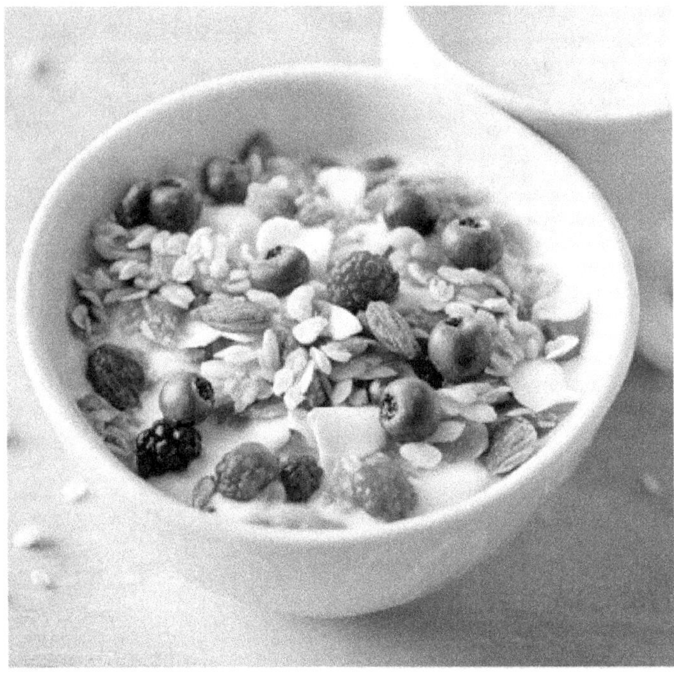

22. Yogurt with Mixed Nuts and Berries

Ingredients:

- 2 cups Greek yogurt
- 1/2 cup mixed nuts (e.g., almonds, walnuts, cashews)
- 1 cup mixed berries (e.g., strawberries, blueberries, raspberries)
- 1 tablespoon honey

Instructions:

1. Divide the Greek yogurt into four bowls.
2. Top each bowl with mixed nuts and mixed berries.
3. Drizzle honey over each serving.
4. Serve immediately.

Nutrition Info per Serving:

- Calories: 250
- Carbohydrates: 25g
- Protein: 15g
- Fat: 10g
- Fiber: 4g
- Sugar: 18g

Number of Servings: 4
Cooking Time: 5 minutes

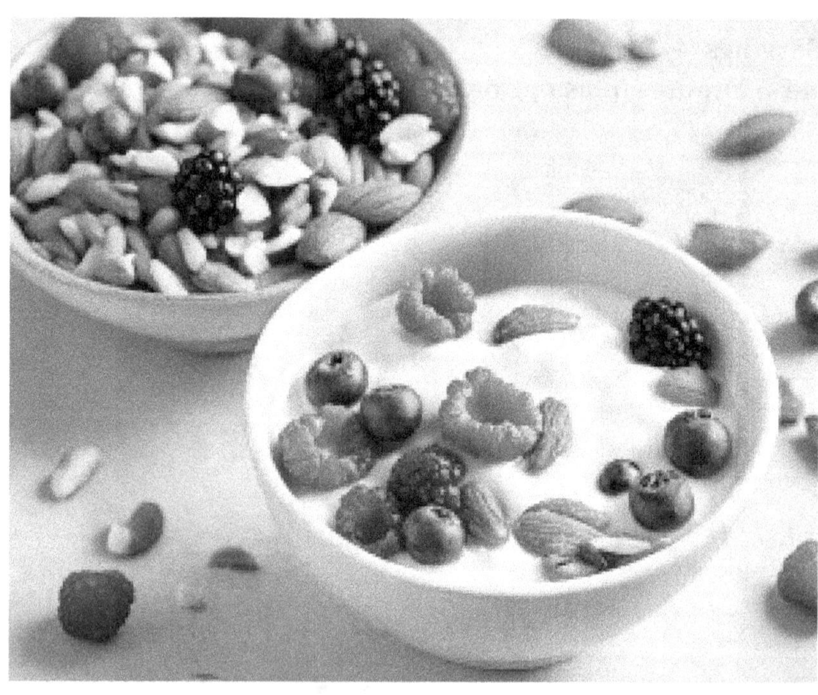

23. Quinoa Porridge

Ingredients:

- 1 cup quinoa, rinsed
- 2 cups water
- 1 cup unsweetened almond milk
- 1 teaspoon cinnamon
- 1/4 teaspoon nutmeg
- 1 tablespoon honey
- 1/2 cup fresh berries

Instructions:

1. In a pot, bring the water to a boil. Add the rinsed quinoa and reduce the heat to a simmer.
2. Cook for 15 minutes or until the water is absorbed.
3. Add the almond milk, cinnamon, nutmeg, and honey. Cook for an additional 5 minutes, stirring frequently, until the porridge is creamy.
4. Serve warm, topped with fresh berries.

Nutrition Info per Serving:

- Calories: 220
- Carbohydrates: 40g
- Protein: 6g
- Fat: 5g
- Fiber: 5g
- Sugar: 12g

Number of Servings: 4
Cooking Time: 25 minutes

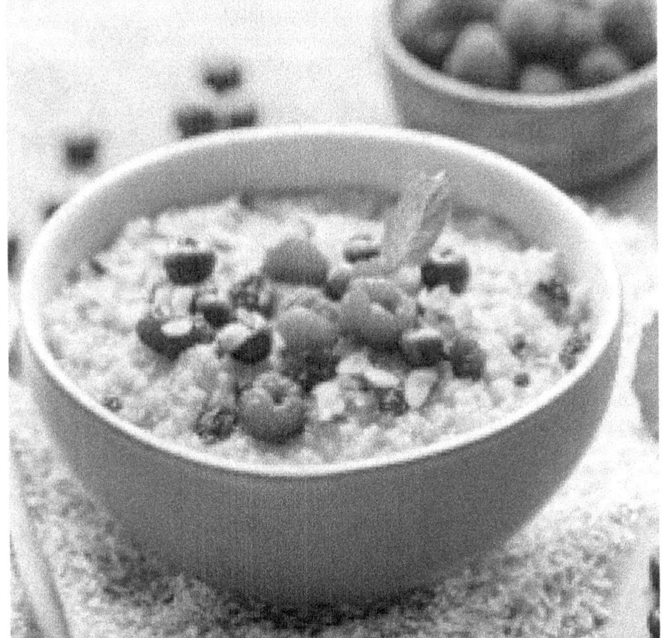

24. Sweet Potato Hash

Ingredients:

- 2 tablespoons olive oil
- 2 medium sweet potatoes, peeled and diced
- 1 small red bell pepper, diced
- 1 small green bell pepper, diced
- 1 small onion, diced
- 2 cloves garlic, minced
- 1/2 teaspoon smoked paprika
- 1/4 teaspoon sea salt
- 1/4 teaspoon black pepper
- 2 tablespoons chopped fresh parsley

Instructions:

1. In a large skillet, heat the olive oil over medium heat.
2. Add the diced sweet potatoes and cook for 10 minutes, stirring occasionally.
3. Add the red bell pepper, green bell pepper, and onion. Cook for another 5 minutes, or until the vegetables are tender.
4. Add the minced garlic, smoked paprika, sea salt, and black pepper. Cook for an additional 2-3 minutes, stirring frequently.
5. Remove from heat and stir in the chopped fresh parsley.
6. Serve warm.

Nutrition Info per Serving:

- Calories: 180
- Carbohydrates: 28g
- Protein: 2g
- Fat: 7g
- Fiber: 5g
- Sugar: 8g

Number of Servings: 4
Cooking Time: 25 minutes

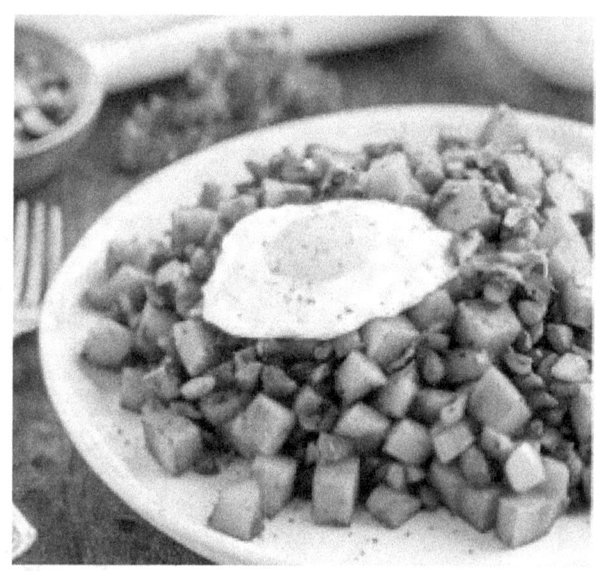

25. Banana Pancakes

Ingredients:

- 1 cup rolled oats
- 1 teaspoon baking powder
- 1/4 teaspoon cinnamon
- 2 ripe bananas
- 2 large eggs
- 1/2 cup unsweetened almond milk
- 1 teaspoon vanilla extract
- 1 tablespoon olive oil (for cooking)
- Fresh berries for topping (optional)
- Maple syrup for serving (optional)

Instructions:

1. In a blender, combine rolled oats, baking powder, and cinnamon. Blend until the oats are finely ground.
2. Add the bananas, eggs, almond milk, and vanilla extract. Blend until smooth.
3. Heat a non-stick skillet or griddle over medium heat and lightly grease with olive oil.
4. Pour 1/4 cup of batter onto the skillet for each pancake. Cook until bubbles form on the surface and the edges look set, about 2-3 minutes. Flip and cook for another 1-2 minutes, until golden brown.
5. Serve warm, topped with fresh berries and maple syrup if desired.

Nutrition Info per Serving (2 pancakes):

- Calories: 180
- Carbohydrates: 30g
- Protein: 5g
- Fat: 5g
- Fiber: 4g
- Sugar: 9g

Number of Servings: 4
Cooking Time: 20 minutes

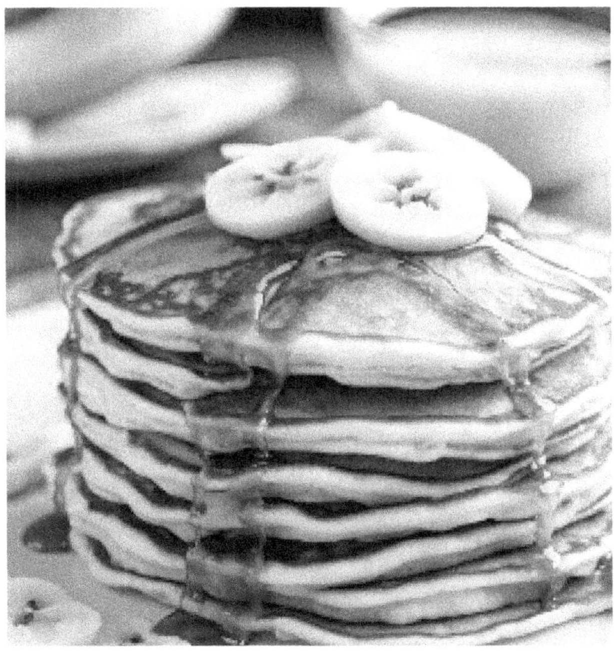

Fish & Seafood Recipes

1. Grilled Salmon with Dill
Ingredients:
- 4 salmon fillets (about 6 ounces each)
- 2 tablespoons olive oil
- 1 tablespoon lemon juice
- 1 tablespoon fresh dill, chopped
- 1 garlic clove, minced
- 1/4 teaspoon sea salt
- 1/4 teaspoon black pepper

Instructions:
1. Preheat the grill to medium-high heat.
2. In a small bowl, mix together olive oil, lemon juice, fresh dill, minced garlic, sea salt, and black pepper.
3. Brush the mixture evenly over the salmon fillets.
4. Place the salmon fillets on the grill, skin-side down.
5. Grill for 5-7 minutes per side, or until the fish flakes easily with a fork.
6. Serve immediately.

Nutrition Info per Serving:
- Calories: 350
- Carbohydrates: 1g
- Protein: 35g
- Fat: 22g
- Fiber: 0g
- Sugar: 0g

Number of Servings: 4
Cooking Time: 15 minutes

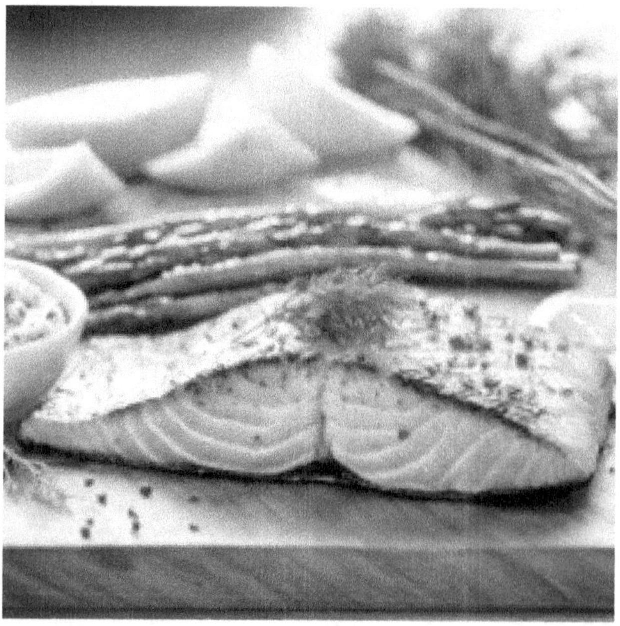

2. Baked Cod with Olive Tapenade

Ingredients:

- 4 cod fillets (about 6 ounces each)
- 1/2 cup pitted Kalamata olives, chopped
- 1/4 cup sun-dried tomatoes, chopped
- 2 tablespoons capers
- 2 tablespoons olive oil
- 1 tablespoon lemon juice
- 1 teaspoon dried oregano
- 1/4 teaspoon sea salt
- 1/4 teaspoon black pepper

Instructions:

1. Preheat the oven to 375°F (190°C).
2. In a small bowl, combine the chopped olives, sun-dried tomatoes, capers, olive oil, lemon juice, dried oregano, sea salt, and black pepper to make the tapenade.
3. Place the cod fillets in a baking dish.
4. Spread the olive tapenade evenly over the cod fillets.
5. Bake for 20-25 minutes, or until the fish flakes easily with a fork.
6. Serve immediately.

Nutrition Info per Serving:

- Calories: 240
- Carbohydrates: 4g
- Protein: 35g
- Fat: 9g
- Fiber: 1g
- Sugar: 2g

Number of Servings: 4
Cooking Time: 30 minutes

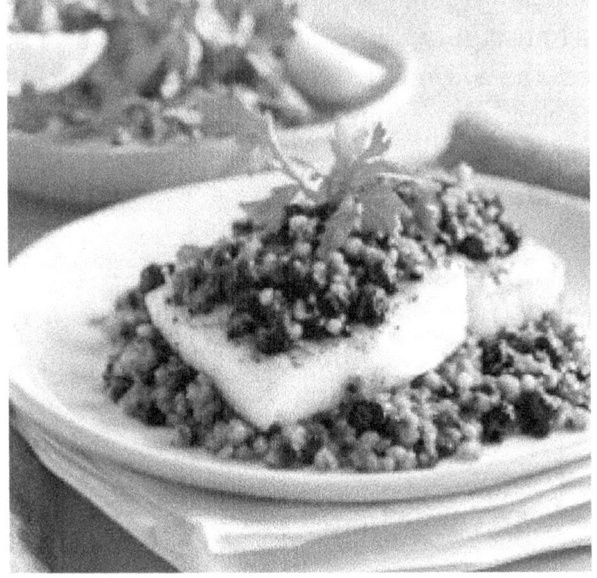

3. Shrimp Stir-Fry with Vegetables

Ingredients:

- 1 pound large shrimp, peeled and deveined
- 2 tablespoons olive oil
- 2 cups broccoli florets
- 1 red bell pepper, sliced
- 1 yellow bell pepper, sliced
- 1 small carrot, thinly sliced
- 2 cloves garlic, minced
- 1 tablespoon fresh ginger, minced
- 2 tablespoons low-sodium soy sauce
- 1 tablespoon rice vinegar
- 1 tablespoon honey
- 1/4 teaspoon red pepper flakes (optional)

Instructions:

1. In a large skillet or wok, heat 1 tablespoon of olive oil over medium-high heat.
2. Add the shrimp and cook for 2-3 minutes on each side, until pink and opaque. Remove from the skillet and set aside.
3. Add the remaining tablespoon of olive oil to the skillet. Add the broccoli, red bell pepper, yellow bell pepper, and carrot. Cook for 5-7 minutes, stirring frequently, until the vegetables are tender-crisp.
4. Add the garlic and ginger, and cook for an additional 1-2 minutes.
5. In a small bowl, mix together the soy sauce, rice vinegar, honey, and red pepper flakes (if using).
6. Return the shrimp to the skillet and pour the sauce over the shrimp and vegetables. Stir to combine and cook for another 2-3 minutes.
7. Serve immediately.

Nutrition Info per Serving:

- Calories: 220
- Carbohydrates: 15g
- Protein: 25g
- Fat: 8g
- Fiber: 3g
- Sugar: 8g

Number of Servings: 4
Cooking Time: 20 minutes

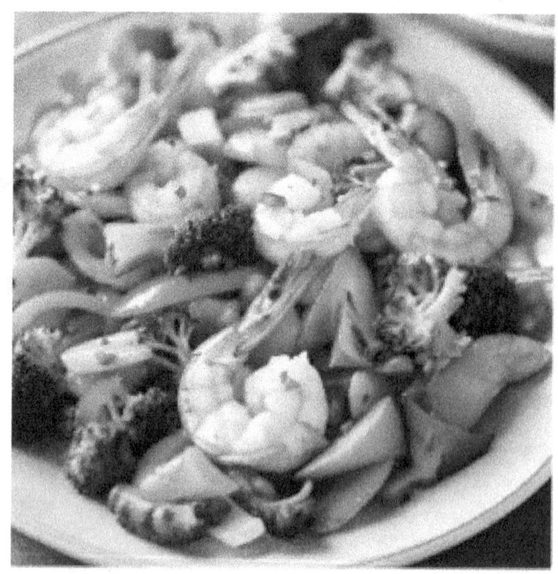

4. Mackerel Salad

Ingredients:

- 2 cans (6 ounces each) mackerel in water, drained and flaked
- 1 cup cherry tomatoes, halved
- 1/2 cucumber, diced
- 1/4 red onion, thinly sliced
- 2 tablespoons capers
- 2 tablespoons fresh parsley, chopped
- 3 tablespoons olive oil
- 1 tablespoon lemon juice
- 1 teaspoon Dijon mustard
- 1/4 teaspoon sea salt
- 1/4 teaspoon black pepper

Instructions:

1. In a large bowl, combine the flaked mackerel, cherry tomatoes, cucumber, red onion, capers, and fresh parsley.
2. In a small bowl, whisk together the olive oil, lemon juice, Dijon mustard, sea salt, and black pepper.
3. Pour the dressing over the mackerel mixture and toss gently to combine.
4. Serve immediately.

Nutrition Info per Serving:

- Calories: 250
- Carbohydrates: 4g
- Protein: 20g
- Fat: 18g
- Fiber: 1g
- Sugar: 2g

Number of Servings: 4
Cooking Time: 10 minutes

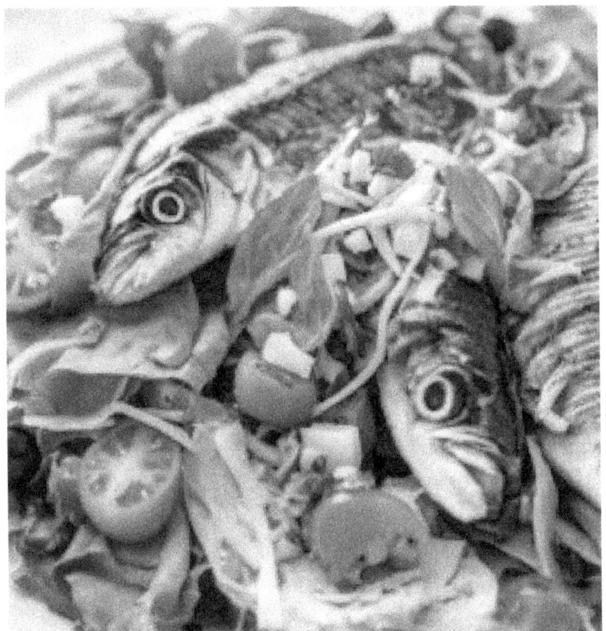

5. Fish Tacos with Cabbage Slaw

Ingredients:

- 1 pound white fish fillets (such as tilapia or cod)
- 2 tablespoons olive oil
- 1 tablespoon lime juice
- 1 teaspoon chili powder
- 1/2 teaspoon cumin
- 1/4 teaspoon sea salt
- 8 small corn tortillas
- 2 cups shredded cabbage
- 1/2 cup shredded carrots
- 1/4 cup chopped fresh cilantro
- 1/4 cup Greek yogurt
- 1 tablespoon lime juice
- 1 teaspoon honey

Instructions:

1. Preheat the grill to medium-high heat.
2. In a small bowl, mix together olive oil, lime juice, chili powder, cumin, and sea salt. Brush the mixture over the fish fillets.
3. Grill the fish for 3-4 minutes per side, until it flakes easily with a fork.
4. In a large bowl, combine shredded cabbage, shredded carrots, and chopped cilantro.
5. In a small bowl, mix together Greek yogurt, lime juice, and honey. Pour over the cabbage mixture and toss to combine.
6. Warm the corn tortillas on the grill for about 30 seconds per side.
7. Fill each tortilla with grilled fish and top with cabbage slaw.
8. Serve immediately.

Nutrition Info per Serving:

- Calories: 250
- Carbohydrates: 25g
- Protein: 20g
- Fat: 10g
- Fiber: 5g
- Sugar: 6g

Number of Servings: 4
Cooking Time: 20 minutes

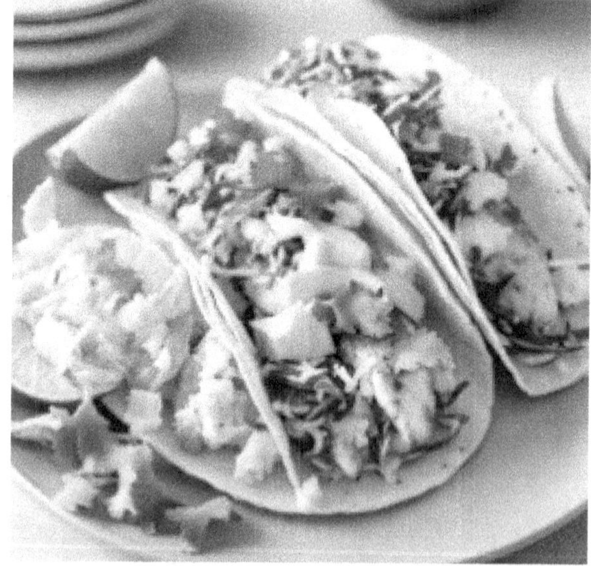

6. Tilapia in Parchment

Ingredients:

- 4 tilapia fillets (about 6 ounces each)
- 1 lemon, thinly sliced
- 1 small zucchini, thinly sliced
- 1 red bell pepper, thinly sliced
- 2 tablespoons olive oil
- 1 teaspoon dried thyme
- 1/4 teaspoon sea salt
- 1/4 teaspoon black pepper
- Parchment paper

Instructions:

1. Preheat the oven to 400°F (200°C).
2. Cut four pieces of parchment paper, each about 15 inches long.
3. Place a tilapia fillet in the center of each piece of parchment paper. Top with lemon slices, zucchini slices, and red bell pepper slices.
4. Drizzle each fillet with olive oil and sprinkle with dried thyme, sea salt, and black pepper.
5. Fold the parchment paper over the fish and vegetables, then fold the edges to seal and create a packet.
6. Place the packets on a baking sheet and bake for 20 minutes.
7. Carefully open the packets and serve immediately.

Nutrition Info per Serving:

- Calories: 230
- Carbohydrates: 8g
- Protein: 30g
- Fat: 10g
- Fiber: 2g
- Sugar: 4g

Number of Servings: 4
Cooking Time: 30 minutes

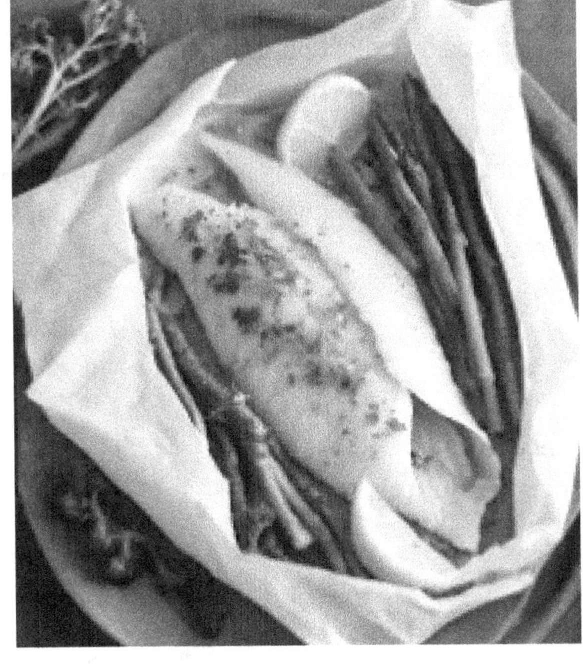

7. Seafood Paella

Ingredients:

- 2 tablespoons olive oil
- 1 onion, diced
- 2 cloves garlic, minced
- 1 red bell pepper, diced
- 1 cup Arborio rice
- 1/4 teaspoon saffron threads
- 1/4 teaspoon smoked paprika
- 4 cups low-sodium chicken or vegetable broth
- 1/2 pound shrimp, peeled and deveined
- 1/2 pound mussels, scrubbed and debearded
- 1/2 pound squid rings
- 1 cup frozen peas, thawed
- 1/4 cup chopped fresh parsley
- 1 lemon, cut into wedges

Instructions:

1. Heat the olive oil in a large skillet or paella pan over medium heat.
2. Add the onion, garlic, and red bell pepper. Cook for 5-7 minutes, until softened.
3. Stir in the Arborio rice, saffron, and smoked paprika. Cook for 2 minutes, stirring constantly.
4. Pour in the broth and bring to a boil. Reduce the heat to low, cover, and simmer for 15 minutes.
5. Add the shrimp, mussels, and squid rings. Cook for another 10 minutes, until the seafood is cooked through and the mussels have opened.
6. Stir in the peas and cook for an additional 2 minutes.
7. Remove from heat and sprinkle with chopped parsley.
8. Serve with lemon wedges.

Nutrition Info per Serving:

- Calories: 350
- Carbohydrates: 40g
- Protein: 30g
- Fat: 10g
- Fiber: 4g
- Sugar: 6g

Number of Servings: 6

Cooking Time: 45 minutes

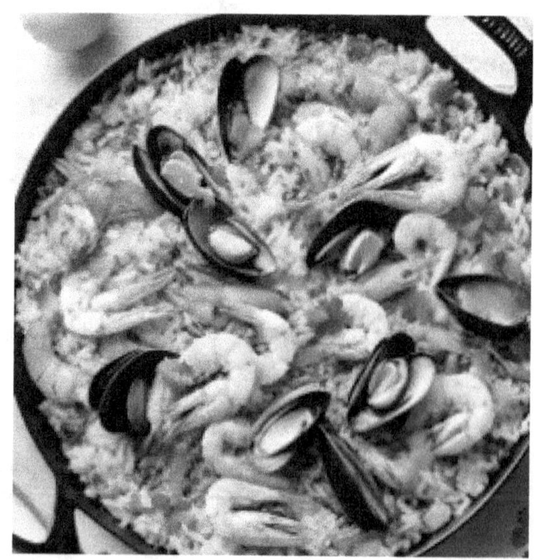

8. Clam Chowder

Ingredients:

- 2 tablespoons olive oil
- 1 onion, diced
- 2 cloves garlic, minced
- 2 celery stalks, diced
- 2 medium potatoes, peeled and diced
- 2 cups low-sodium vegetable broth
- 2 cups unsweetened almond milk
- 1 pound fresh clams, scrubbed and debearded
- 1/2 teaspoon dried thyme
- 1/4 teaspoon sea salt
- 1/4 teaspoon black pepper
- 1/4 cup chopped fresh parsley

Instructions:

1. Heat the olive oil in a large pot over medium heat.
2. Add the onion, garlic, and celery. Cook for 5-7 minutes, until softened.
3. Add the diced potatoes and vegetable broth. Bring to a boil, then reduce the heat and simmer for 15 minutes, until the potatoes are tender.
4. Stir in the almond milk, clams, dried thyme, sea salt, and black pepper. Cook for another 10 minutes, until the clams have opened.
5. Remove from heat and sprinkle with chopped fresh parsley.
6. Serve immediately.

Nutrition Info per Serving:

- Calories: 250
- Carbohydrates: 30g
- Protein: 20g
- Fat: 8g
- Fiber: 4g
- Sugar: 4g

Number of Servings: 4
Cooking Time: 35 minutes

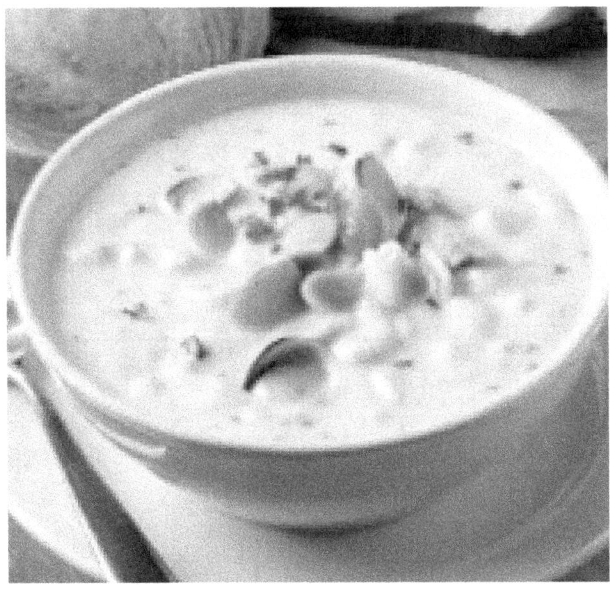

9. Grilled Tuna Steak

Ingredients:

- 4 tuna steaks (about 6 ounces each)
- 2 tablespoons olive oil
- 1 tablespoon lemon juice
- 1 teaspoon dried oregano
- 1/4 teaspoon sea salt
- 1/4 teaspoon black pepper

Instructions:

1. Preheat the grill to high heat.
2. In a small bowl, mix together olive oil, lemon juice, dried oregano, sea salt, and black pepper.
3. Brush the mixture over both sides of the tuna steaks.
4. Grill the tuna steaks for 2-3 minutes per side, until seared on the outside but still pink in the center.
5. Serve immediately.

Nutrition Info per Serving:

- Calories: 300
- Carbohydrates: 1g
- Protein: 35g
- Fat: 18g
- Fiber: 0g
- Sugar: 0g

Number of Servings: 4
Cooking Time: 10 minutes

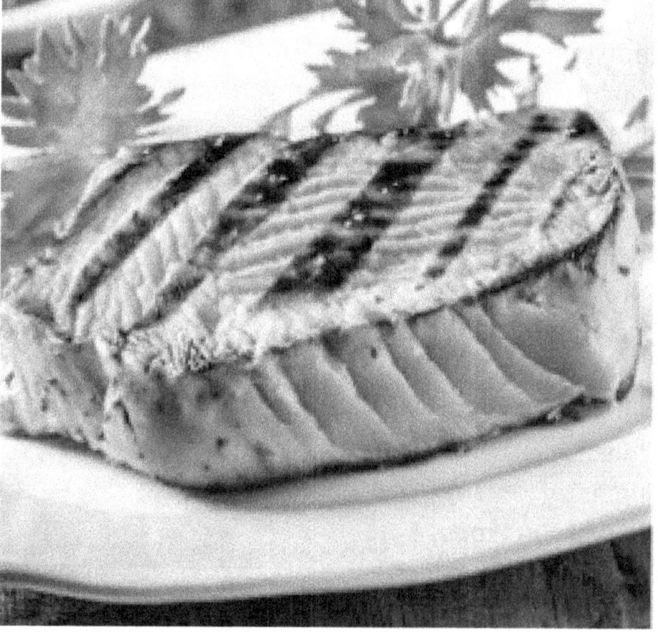

10. Seafood Gumbo

Ingredients:

- 3 tablespoons olive oil
- 1/4 cup whole wheat flour
- 1 onion, diced
- 1 green bell pepper, diced
- 2 celery stalks, diced
- 2 cloves garlic, minced
- 4 cups low-sodium chicken or vegetable broth
- 1 can (14.5 ounces) diced tomatoes
- 1 teaspoon dried thyme
- 1 teaspoon smoked paprika
- 1/2 teaspoon cayenne pepper
- 1/2 teaspoon sea salt
- 1/4 teaspoon black pepper
- 1/2 pound shrimp, peeled and deveined
- 1/2 pound crab meat
- 1/2 pound firm white fish (such as cod or halibut), cut into chunks
- 1/2 cup sliced okra
- 1/4 cup chopped fresh parsley
- 2 cups cooked brown rice (for serving)

Instructions:

1. In a large pot, heat the olive oil over medium heat. Add the whole wheat flour and cook, stirring constantly, until it turns a light brown color (about 5 minutes).
2. Add the onion, green bell pepper, celery, and garlic. Cook for 5-7 minutes, until softened.
3. Stir in the broth, diced tomatoes, dried thyme, smoked paprika, cayenne pepper, sea salt, and black pepper. Bring to a boil, then reduce the heat and simmer for 20 minutes.
4. Add the shrimp, crab meat, white fish, and okra. Cook for another 10 minutes, until the seafood is cooked through.
5. Remove from heat and stir in the chopped fresh parsley.
6. Serve over cooked brown rice.

Nutrition Info per Serving:

- Calories: 400
- Carbohydrates: 40g
- Protein: 30g
- Fat: 12g
- Fiber: 5g
- Sugar: 6g

Number of Servings: 6
Cooking Time: 45 minutes

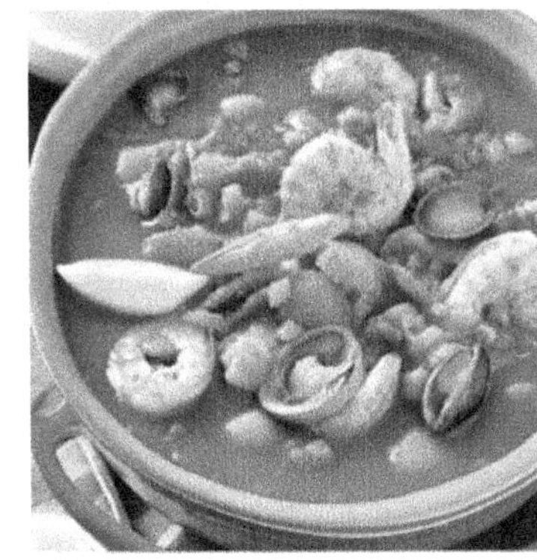

11. Pesto Halibut

Ingredients:

- 4 halibut fillets (about 6 ounces each)
- 1/2 cup prepared basil pesto
- 1 tablespoon olive oil
- 1 tablespoon lemon juice
- 1/4 teaspoon sea salt
- 1/4 teaspoon black pepper

Instructions:

1. Preheat the oven to 400°F (200°C).
2. Place the halibut fillets in a baking dish.
3. In a small bowl, mix together the basil pesto, olive oil, lemon juice, sea salt, and black pepper.
4. Spread the pesto mixture evenly over the halibut fillets.
5. Bake for 15-20 minutes, or until the fish flakes easily with a fork.
6. Serve immediately.

Nutrition Info per Serving:

- Calories: 300
- Carbohydrates: 2g
- Protein: 34g
- Fat: 18g
- Fiber: 1g
- Sugar: 0g

Number of Servings: 4
Cooking Time: 25 minutes

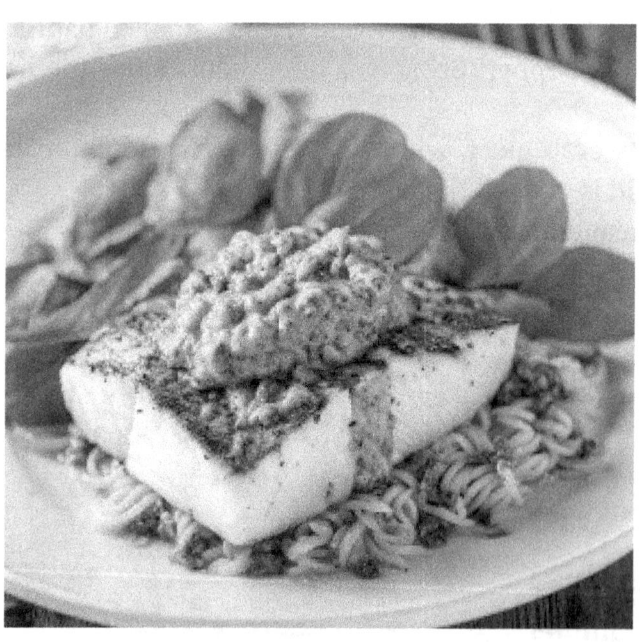

12. Crab Cakes

Ingredients:

- 1 pound lump crab meat
- 1/2 cup whole wheat breadcrumbs
- 1/4 cup Greek yogurt
- 1 egg, beaten
- 1 tablespoon Dijon mustard
- 1 tablespoon lemon juice
- 1 tablespoon fresh parsley, chopped
- 1 teaspoon Old Bay seasoning
- 1/4 teaspoon sea salt
- 2 tablespoons olive oil (for cooking)

Instructions:

1. In a large bowl, combine crab meat, whole wheat breadcrumbs, Greek yogurt, beaten egg, Dijon mustard, lemon juice, fresh parsley, Old Bay seasoning, and sea salt.
2. Form the mixture into 8 patties.
3. Heat the olive oil in a large skillet over medium heat.
4. Cook the crab cakes for 3-4 minutes per side, until golden brown and cooked through.
5. Serve immediately.

Nutrition Info per Serving (2 crab cakes):

- Calories: 250
- Carbohydrates: 10g
- Protein: 26g
- Fat: 12g
- Fiber: 2g
- Sugar: 2g

Number of Servings: 4
Cooking Time: 20 minutes

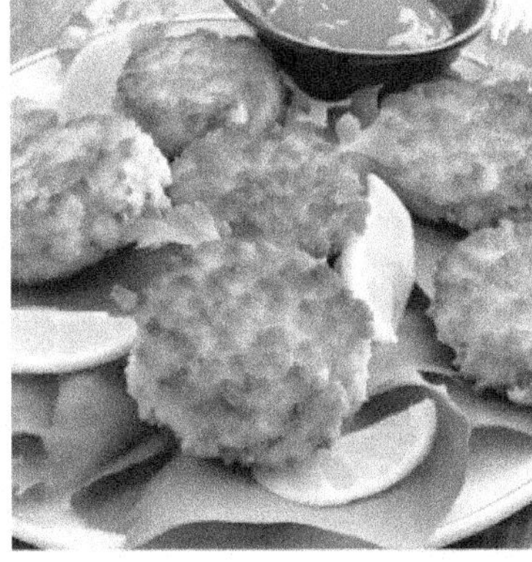

13. Cajun Catfish
Ingredients:
- 4 catfish fillets (about 6 ounces each)
- 2 tablespoons olive oil
- 1 tablespoon Cajun seasoning
- 1 tablespoon lemon juice
- 1/4 teaspoon sea salt
- 1/4 teaspoon black pepper

Instructions:
1. Preheat the grill to medium-high heat.
2. In a small bowl, mix together olive oil, Cajun seasoning, lemon juice, sea salt, and black pepper.
3. Brush the mixture evenly over the catfish fillets.
4. Grill the catfish for 3-4 minutes per side, until it flakes easily with a fork.
5. Serve immediately.

Nutrition Info per Serving:
- Calories: 250
- Carbohydrates: 1g
- Protein: 30g
- Fat: 14g
- Fiber: 0g
- Sugar: 0g

Number of Servings: 4
Cooking Time: 15 minutes

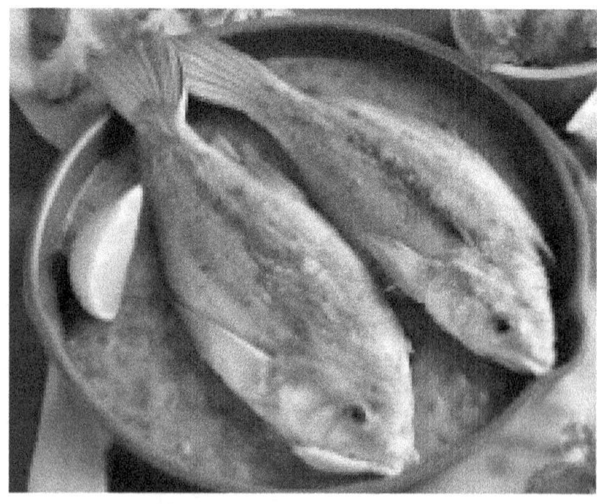

14. Haddock in Tomato Basil Sauce

Ingredients:

- 4 haddock fillets (about 6 ounces each)
- 2 tablespoons olive oil
- 1 onion, diced
- 2 cloves garlic, minced
- 1 can (14.5 ounces) diced tomatoes
- 1/4 cup tomato paste
- 1/2 cup fresh basil, chopped
- 1/4 teaspoon sea salt
- 1/4 teaspoon black pepper

Instructions:

1. Preheat the oven to 375°F (190°C).
2. Heat the olive oil in a large skillet over medium heat.
3. Add the onion and garlic. Cook for 5-7 minutes, until softened.
4. Stir in the diced tomatoes, tomato paste, fresh basil, sea salt, and black pepper. Cook for another 5 minutes.
5. Place the haddock fillets in a baking dish. Pour the tomato basil sauce over the fish.
6. Bake for 20-25 minutes, or until the fish flakes easily with a fork.
7. Serve immediately.

Nutrition Info per Serving:

- Calories: 220
- Carbohydrates: 10g
- Protein: 30g
- Fat: 8g
- Fiber: 2g
- Sugar: 6g

Number of Servings: 4
Cooking Time: 30 minutes

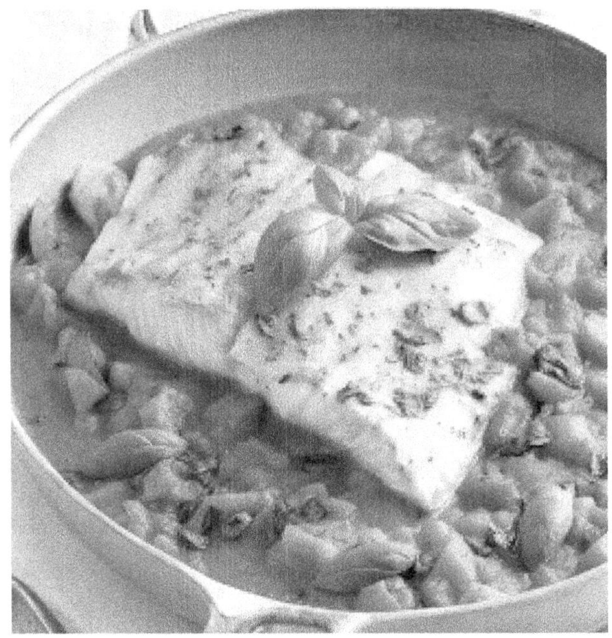

15. Fish Curry

Ingredients:

- 1 tablespoon olive oil
- 1 onion, diced
- 2 cloves garlic, minced
- 1 tablespoon fresh ginger, minced
- 1 tablespoon curry powder
- 1 teaspoon turmeric
- 1 can (14.5 ounces) coconut milk
- 1 can (14.5 ounces) diced tomatoes
- 1 pound firm white fish (such as cod or halibut), cut into chunks
- 1/2 cup peas (fresh or frozen)
- 1/4 cup fresh cilantro, chopped
- 1/4 teaspoon sea salt
- 1/4 teaspoon black pepper
- 1 lime, cut into wedges

Instructions:

1. Heat the olive oil in a large pot over medium heat.
2. Add the onion, garlic, and ginger. Cook for 5-7 minutes, until softened.
3. Stir in the curry powder and turmeric. Cook for 1 minute, until fragrant.
4. Add the coconut milk and diced tomatoes. Bring to a simmer.
5. Add the fish chunks and peas. Cook for 10 minutes, until the fish is cooked through.
6. Remove from heat and stir in the fresh cilantro.
7. Serve with lime wedges.

Nutrition Info per Serving:

- Calories: 300
- Carbohydrates: 12g
- Protein: 28g
- Fat: 16g
- Fiber: 3g
- Sugar: 7g

Number of Servings: 4
Cooking Time: 25 minutes

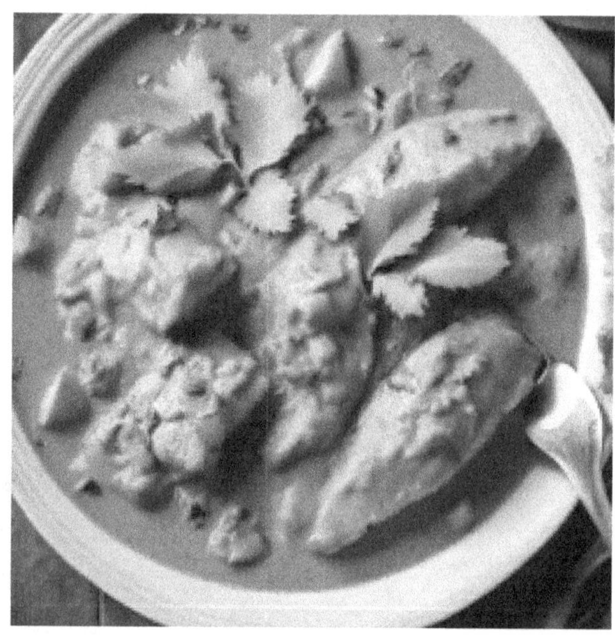

16. Oysters Rockefeller

Ingredients:

- 12 fresh oysters, shucked
- 1 tablespoon olive oil
- 2 cloves garlic, minced
- 2 cups fresh spinach, chopped
- 1/4 cup breadcrumbs (whole wheat or gluten-free)
- 1/4 cup Parmesan cheese, grated
- 1/4 teaspoon sea salt
- 1/4 teaspoon black pepper
- 1 tablespoon fresh lemon juice

Instructions:

1. Preheat the oven to 450°F (230°C).
2. Arrange the oysters on a baking sheet.
3. Heat the olive oil in a skillet over medium heat. Add the garlic and spinach. Cook for 3-4 minutes, until the spinach is wilted.
4. In a small bowl, combine the breadcrumbs, Parmesan cheese, sea salt, and black pepper.
5. Top each oyster with a spoonful of the spinach mixture, then sprinkle with the breadcrumb mixture.
6. Bake for 10-12 minutes, until the topping is golden brown.
7. Drizzle with fresh lemon juice before serving.

Nutrition Info per Serving:

- Calories: 180
- Carbohydrates: 8g
- Protein: 14g
- Fat: 10g
- Fiber: 1g
- Sugar: 1g

Number of Servings: 4
Cooking Time: 20 minutes

17. Trout Almondine

Ingredients:

- 4 trout fillets (about 6 ounces each)
- 1/4 cup whole wheat flour
- 2 tablespoons olive oil
- 1/4 cup sliced almonds
- 2 tablespoons fresh lemon juice
- 2 tablespoons fresh parsley, chopped
- 1/4 teaspoon sea salt
- 1/4 teaspoon black pepper

Instructions:

1. Preheat the oven to 350°F (175°C).
2. Lightly coat the trout fillets with whole wheat flour.
3. In a large skillet, heat the olive oil over medium heat. Add the trout fillets and cook for 3-4 minutes on each side, until golden brown.
4. Transfer the trout fillets to a baking dish and place in the oven to keep warm.
5. In the same skillet, add the sliced almonds and cook for 2-3 minutes, until golden and fragrant.
6. Remove from heat and stir in the lemon juice, fresh parsley, sea salt, and black pepper.
7. Pour the almond mixture over the trout fillets.
8. Serve immediately.

Nutrition Info per Serving:

- Calories: 280
- Carbohydrates: 6g
- Protein: 28g
- Fat: 16g
- Fiber: 2g
- Sugar: 1g

Number of Servings: 4

Cooking Time: 20 minutes

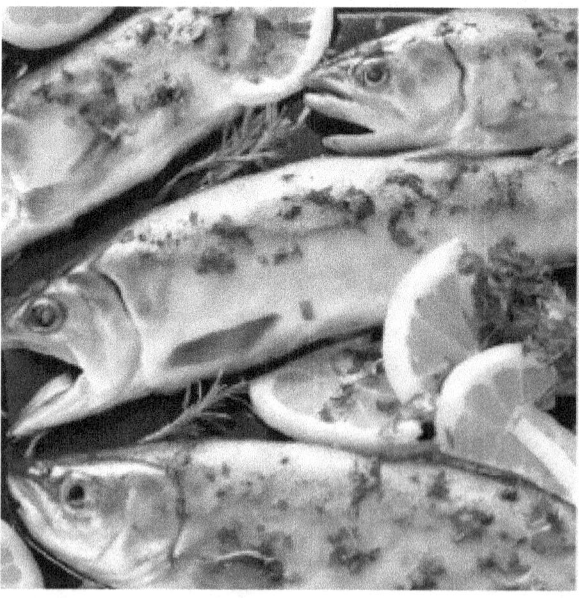

18. Scallop Pasta with Asparagus

Ingredients:

- 8 ounces whole wheat pasta
- 1 pound sea scallops
- 2 tablespoons olive oil
- 2 cloves garlic, minced
- 1 bunch asparagus, trimmed and cut into 1-inch pieces
- 1/4 cup low-sodium chicken broth
- 1/4 cup fresh lemon juice
- 1/4 cup grated Parmesan cheese
- 1/4 teaspoon sea salt
- 1/4 teaspoon black pepper
- 1/4 cup fresh parsley, chopped

Instructions:

1. Cook the pasta according to package instructions. Drain and set aside.
2. Pat the scallops dry and season with sea salt and black pepper.
3. In a large skillet, heat 1 tablespoon of olive oil over medium-high heat. Add the scallops and cook for 2-3 minutes on each side, until golden brown. Remove from the skillet and set aside.
4. In the same skillet, heat the remaining tablespoon of olive oil over medium heat. Add the garlic and asparagus, and cook for 5-7 minutes, until the asparagus is tender.
5. Stir in the chicken broth and lemon juice, and cook for an additional 2 minutes.
6. Add the cooked pasta and scallops back to the skillet, and toss to combine.
7. Sprinkle with Parmesan cheese and fresh parsley.
8. Serve immediately.

Nutrition Info per Serving:

- Calories: 380
- Carbohydrates: 45g
- Protein: 28g
- Fat: 12g
- Fiber: 7g
- Sugar: 4g

Number of Servings: 4

Cooking Time: 30 minutes

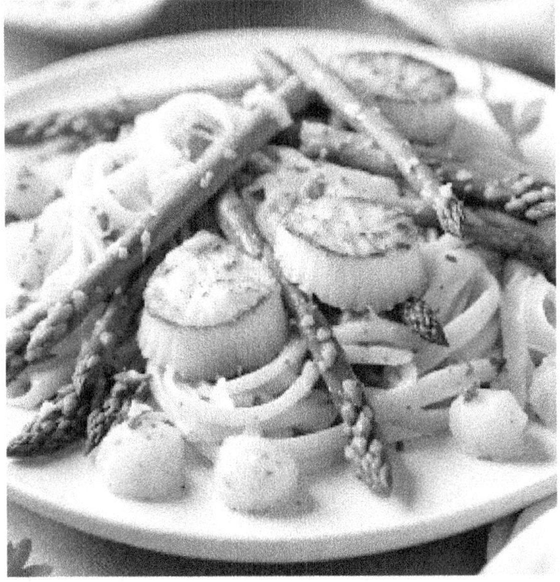

19. Grilled Mahi Mahi with Mango Salsa

Ingredients:

- 4 mahi mahi fillets (about 6 ounces each)
- 2 tablespoons olive oil
- 1 tablespoon lime juice
- 1 teaspoon ground cumin
- 1/4 teaspoon sea salt
- 1/4 teaspoon black pepper
- 1 ripe mango, peeled and diced
- 1/2 red bell pepper, diced
- 1/4 red onion, finely chopped
- 1/4 cup fresh cilantro, chopped
- 1 tablespoon lime juice

Instructions:

1. Preheat the grill to medium-high heat.
2. In a small bowl, mix together olive oil, lime juice, ground cumin, sea salt, and black pepper. Brush the mixture over the mahi mahi fillets.
3. Grill the fillets for 4-5 minutes on each side, until the fish flakes easily with a fork.
4. In a medium bowl, combine the diced mango, red bell pepper, red onion, cilantro, and lime juice.
5. Serve the grilled mahi mahi topped with mango salsa.

Nutrition Info per Serving:

- Calories: 320
- Carbohydrates: 15g
- Protein: 34g
- Fat: 14g
- Fiber: 3g
- Sugar: 10g

Number of Servings: 4
Cooking Time: 20 minutes

20. Shrimp and Broccoli Alfredo

Ingredients:

- 8 ounces whole wheat fettuccine
- 1 pound large shrimp, peeled and deveined
- 2 tablespoons olive oil
- 3 cups broccoli florets
- 3 cloves garlic, minced
- 1 cup unsweetened almond milk
- 1/2 cup grated Parmesan cheese
- 1/4 teaspoon sea salt
- 1/4 teaspoon black pepper
- 1/4 teaspoon nutmeg
- 1/4 cup fresh parsley, chopped

Instructions:

1. Cook the fettuccine according to package instructions. Drain and set aside.
2. In a large skillet, heat 1 tablespoon of olive oil over medium heat. Add the shrimp and cook for 2-3 minutes on each side, until pink and opaque. Remove from the skillet and set aside.
3. In the same skillet, heat the remaining tablespoon of olive oil over medium heat. Add the broccoli and garlic, and cook for 5-7 minutes, until the broccoli is tender.
4. Stir in the almond milk, Parmesan cheese, sea salt, black pepper, and nutmeg. Cook for 2-3 minutes, until the sauce thickens slightly.
5. Add the cooked fettuccine and shrimp back to the skillet, and toss to combine.
6. Sprinkle with fresh parsley.
7. Serve immediately.

Nutrition Info per Serving:

- Calories: 380
- Carbohydrates: 45g
- Protein: 28g
- Fat: 12g
- Fiber: 7g
- Sugar: 4g

Number of Servings: 4
Cooking Time: 30 minutes

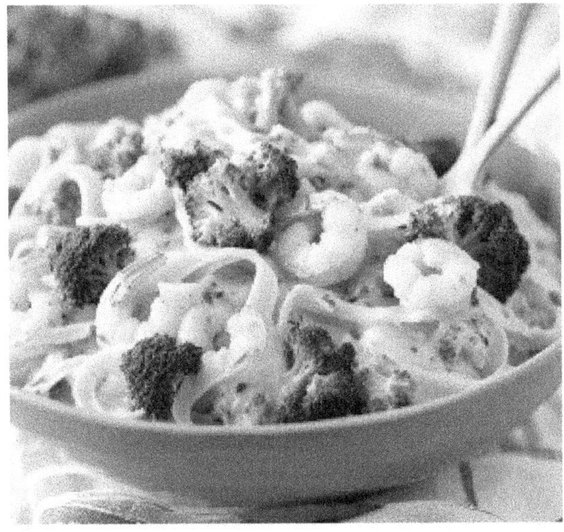

21. Salmon and Spinach Quiche

Ingredients:

- 1 whole wheat pie crust
- 1 cup cooked salmon, flaked
- 1 cup fresh spinach, chopped
- 1/2 cup onion, finely chopped
- 1 cup low-fat milk
- 4 large eggs
- 1/2 cup grated Parmesan cheese
- 1/4 teaspoon sea salt
- 1/4 teaspoon black pepper

Instructions:

1. Preheat the oven to 375°F (190°C).
2. Place the whole wheat pie crust in a pie dish and set aside.
3. In a large bowl, whisk together the eggs, milk, sea salt, and black pepper.
4. Layer the flaked salmon, chopped spinach, and onion evenly in the pie crust.
5. Pour the egg mixture over the salmon and spinach, then sprinkle the grated Parmesan cheese on top.
6. Bake for 35-40 minutes, or until the quiche is set and the top is golden brown.
7. Allow to cool for a few minutes before slicing and serving.

Nutrition Info per Serving:

- Calories: 250
- Carbohydrates: 15g
- Protein: 18g
- Fat: 14g
- Fiber: 2g
- Sugar: 3g

Number of Servings: 6
Cooking Time: 45 minutes

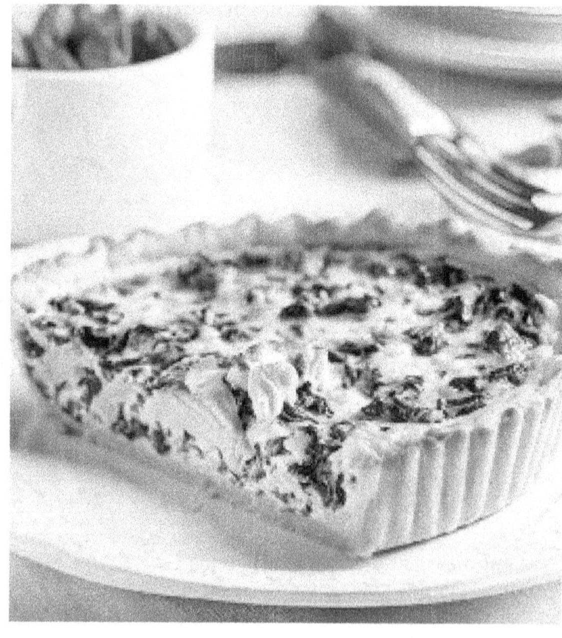

22. Fish Stew with Vegetables

Ingredients:

- 1 tablespoon olive oil
- 1 onion, diced
- 2 cloves garlic, minced
- 2 celery stalks, diced
- 2 carrots, sliced
- 1 red bell pepper, diced
- 1 can (14.5 ounces) diced tomatoes
- 4 cups low-sodium vegetable broth
- 1 pound firm white fish (such as cod or halibut), cut into chunks
- 1/2 teaspoon dried thyme
- 1/4 teaspoon sea salt
- 1/4 teaspoon black pepper
- 1/4 cup fresh parsley, chopped

Instructions:

1. Heat the olive oil in a large pot over medium heat.
2. Add the onion, garlic, celery, carrots, and red bell pepper. Cook for 5-7 minutes, until softened.
3. Stir in the diced tomatoes, vegetable broth, dried thyme, sea salt, and black pepper. Bring to a simmer.
4. Add the fish chunks and cook for 10-12 minutes, until the fish is cooked through.
5. Remove from heat and stir in the fresh parsley.
6. Serve immediately.

Nutrition Info per Serving:

- Calories: 220
- Carbohydrates: 15g
- Protein: 25g
- Fat: 7g
- Fiber: 4g
- Sugar: 7g

Number of Servings: 4
Cooking Time: 35 minutes

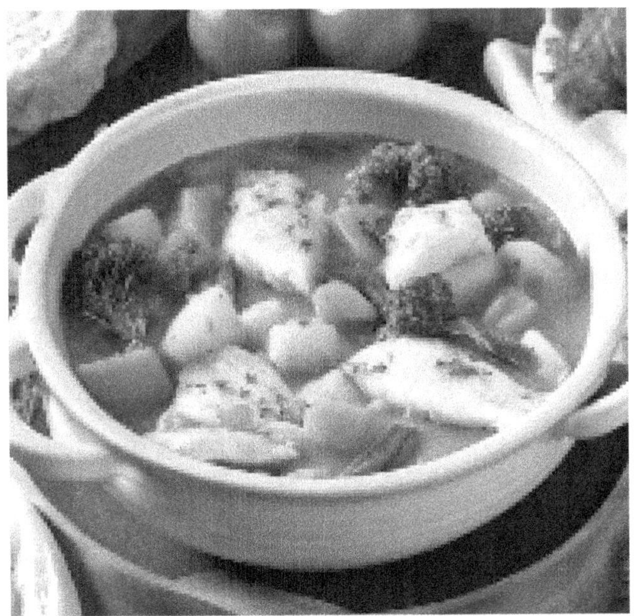

23. Spicy Tuna Rolls

Ingredients:

- 1 cup sushi rice
- 2 tablespoons rice vinegar
- 1 teaspoon honey
- 1/2 teaspoon sea salt
- 4 sheets nori (seaweed)
- 1/2 pound fresh tuna, finely chopped
- 1 tablespoon Sriracha sauce
- 1 small cucumber, julienned
- 1 avocado, sliced
- 2 tablespoons sesame seeds

Instructions:

1. Cook the sushi rice according to package instructions. Stir in the rice vinegar, honey, and sea salt. Let the rice cool.
2. In a small bowl, mix the chopped tuna with Sriracha sauce.
3. Place a sheet of nori on a bamboo sushi mat. Spread 1/4 of the rice evenly over the nori, leaving a 1-inch border at the top.
4. Arrange some cucumber, avocado, and spicy tuna mixture along the bottom edge of the rice.
5. Roll the nori tightly around the filling using the bamboo mat, sealing the edge with a bit of water.
6. Repeat with the remaining ingredients to make four rolls.
7. Slice each roll into 8 pieces and sprinkle with sesame seeds.
8. Serve immediately.

Nutrition Info per Serving (8 pieces):

- Calories: 250
- Carbohydrates: 28g
- Protein: 15g
- Fat: 9g
- Fiber: 4g
- Sugar: 4g

Number of Servings: 4
Cooking Time: 40 minutes

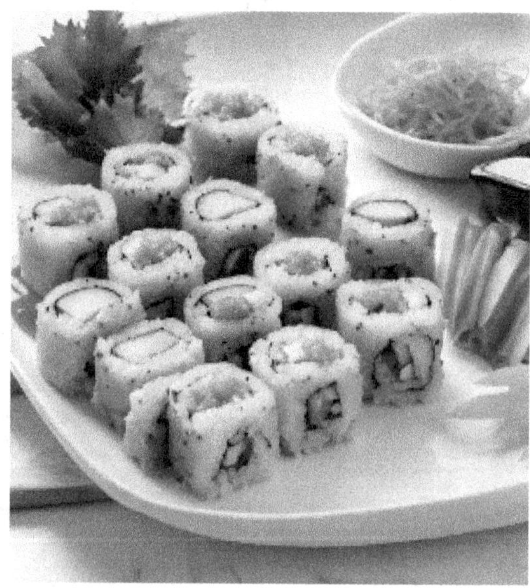

24. Baked Snapper with Citrus

Ingredients:

- 4 snapper fillets (about 6 ounces each)
- 2 tablespoons olive oil
- 1 orange, thinly sliced
- 1 lemon, thinly sliced
- 1 lime, thinly sliced
- 1 teaspoon dried oregano
- 1/4 teaspoon sea salt
- 1/4 teaspoon black pepper

Instructions:

1. Preheat the oven to 375°F (190°C).
2. Place the snapper fillets in a baking dish.
3. Drizzle the olive oil over the fish and sprinkle with dried oregano, sea salt, and black pepper.
4. Arrange the orange, lemon, and lime slices over the fish.
5. Bake for 20-25 minutes, or until the fish flakes easily with a fork.
6. Serve immediately.

Nutrition Info per Serving:

- Calories: 280
- Carbohydrates: 8g
- Protein: 30g
- Fat: 14g
- Fiber: 2g
- Sugar: 3g

Number of Servings: 4
Cooking Time: 30 minutes

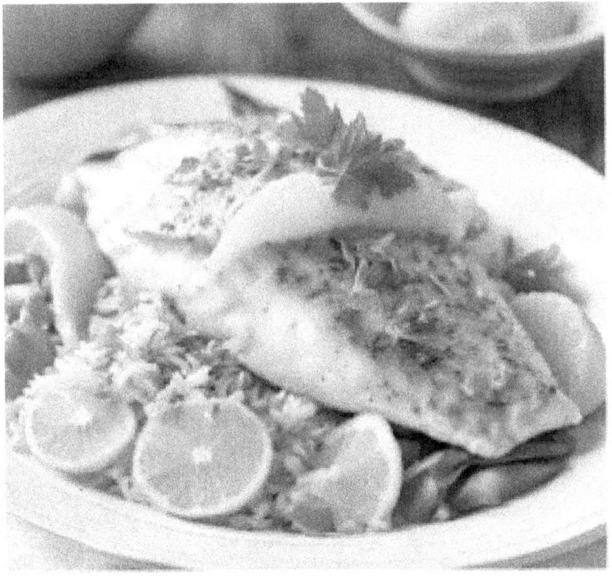

25. Sea Bass with Ginger Soy Glaze
Ingredients:

- 4 sea bass fillets (about 6 ounces each)
- 2 tablespoons olive oil
- 1/4 cup low-sodium soy sauce
- 2 tablespoons honey
- 1 tablespoon fresh ginger, grated
- 2 cloves garlic, minced
- 1/4 teaspoon sea salt
- 1/4 teaspoon black pepper
- 1/4 cup green onions, chopped

Instructions:

1. Preheat the oven to 375°F (190°C).
2. In a small bowl, mix together the soy sauce, honey, grated ginger, minced garlic, sea salt, and black pepper.
3. Place the sea bass fillets in a baking dish and pour the ginger soy glaze over the fish.
4. Drizzle the olive oil over the fillets.
5. Bake for 20-25 minutes, or until the fish flakes easily with a fork.
6. Sprinkle with chopped green onions before serving.
7. Serve immediately.

Nutrition Info per Serving:

- Calories: 310
- Carbohydrates: 10g
- Protein: 32g
- Fat: 16g
- Fiber: 1g
- Sugar: 6g

Number of Servings: 4
Cooking Time: 30 minutes

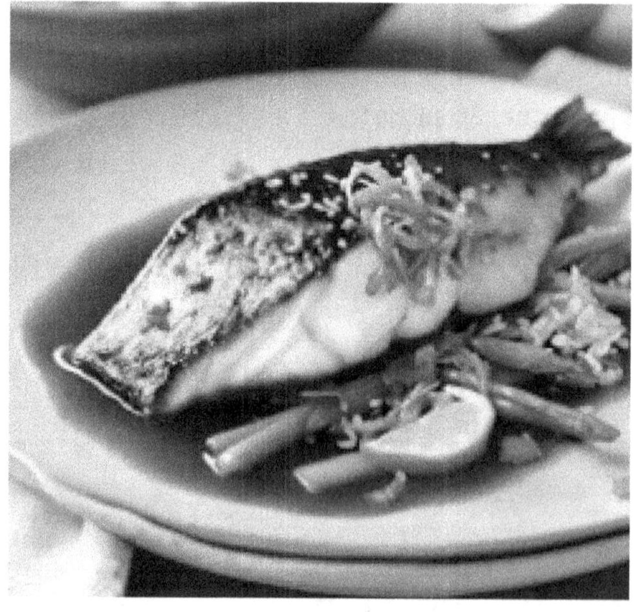

Poultry Recipes

1. Grilled Chicken Salad

Ingredients:

- 2 boneless, skinless chicken breasts
- 2 tablespoons olive oil
- 1 tablespoon lemon juice
- 1 teaspoon dried oregano
- 1/4 teaspoon sea salt
- 1/4 teaspoon black pepper
- 6 cups mixed greens (spinach, arugula, lettuce)
- 1 cup cherry tomatoes, halved
- 1/2 cucumber, sliced
- 1/4 red onion, thinly sliced
- 1/4 cup feta cheese, crumbled
- 1/4 cup olives, pitted and sliced

Instructions:

1. Preheat the grill to medium-high heat.
2. In a small bowl, mix together olive oil, lemon juice, dried oregano, sea salt, and black pepper.
3. Brush the mixture over the chicken breasts.
4. Grill the chicken for 6-7 minutes on each side, or until cooked through and the internal temperature reaches 165°F (74°C).
5. Remove from the grill and let it rest for 5 minutes before slicing.
6. In a large bowl, combine mixed greens, cherry tomatoes, cucumber, red onion, feta cheese, and olives.
7. Top the salad with sliced grilled chicken.
8. Serve immediately.

Nutrition Info per Serving:

- Calories: 320
- Carbohydrates: 10g
- Protein: 34g
- Fat: 18g
- Fiber: 3g
- Sugar: 4g

Number of Servings: 4
Cooking Time: 20 minutes

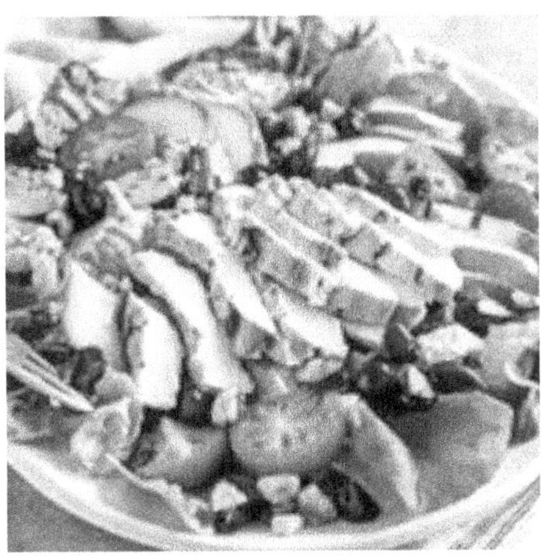

2. Turmeric Chicken Soup
Ingredients:

- 1 tablespoon olive oil
- 1 onion, diced
- 2 cloves garlic, minced
- 2 carrots, sliced
- 2 celery stalks, sliced
- 1 pound boneless, skinless chicken thighs, cut into bite-sized pieces
- 1 teaspoon ground turmeric
- 1 teaspoon ground ginger
- 6 cups low-sodium chicken broth
- 1 cup kale, chopped
- 1/2 teaspoon sea salt
- 1/4 teaspoon black pepper
- 1 tablespoon fresh lemon juice

Instructions:

1. Heat the olive oil in a large pot over medium heat.
2. Add the onion, garlic, carrots, and celery. Cook for 5-7 minutes, until softened.
3. Add the chicken pieces and cook for another 5 minutes, until the chicken is lightly browned.
4. Stir in the ground turmeric and ground ginger. Cook for 1 minute.
5. Pour in the chicken broth and bring to a boil. Reduce the heat and simmer for 20 minutes.
6. Add the chopped kale and cook for an additional 5 minutes.
7. Stir in the sea salt, black pepper, and fresh lemon juice.
8. Serve immediately.

Nutrition Info per Serving:

- Calories: 220
- Carbohydrates: 10g
- Protein: 26g
- Fat: 10g
- Fiber: 3g
- Sugar: 4g

Number of Servings: 6
Cooking Time: 35 minutes

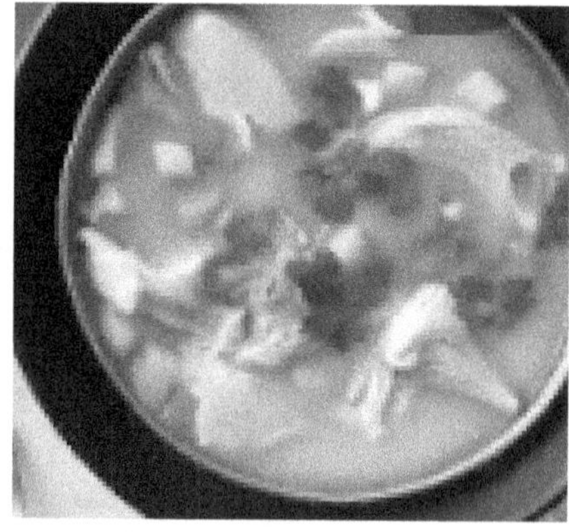

3. Rosemary Lemon Roast Chicken

Ingredients:

- 1 whole chicken (about 4 pounds)
- 2 tablespoons olive oil
- 2 lemons, sliced
- 4 sprigs fresh rosemary
- 4 cloves garlic, minced
- 1 teaspoon sea salt
- 1/2 teaspoon black pepper

Instructions:

1. Preheat the oven to 375°F (190°C).
2. Place the chicken in a roasting pan.
3. In a small bowl, mix together olive oil, minced garlic, sea salt, and black pepper.
4. Rub the mixture all over the chicken, including under the skin.
5. Stuff the cavity of the chicken with lemon slices and rosemary sprigs.
6. Arrange the remaining lemon slices around the chicken in the roasting pan.
7. Roast for 1 hour and 20 minutes, or until the internal temperature reaches 165°F (74°C) and the juices run clear.
8. Let the chicken rest for 10 minutes before carving.
9. Serve immediately.

Nutrition Info per Serving:

- Calories: 350
- Carbohydrates: 2g
- Protein: 40g
- Fat: 20g
- Fiber: 1g
- Sugar: 0g

Number of Servings: 6
Cooking Time: 90 minutes

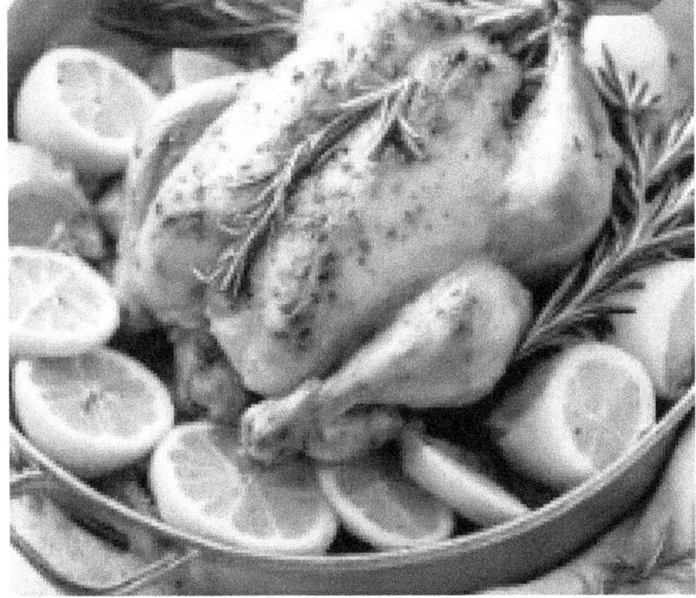

4. Turkey Meatballs in Tomato Sauce

Ingredients:

- 1 pound ground turkey
- 1/4 cup whole wheat breadcrumbs
- 1/4 cup grated Parmesan cheese
- 1 egg, beaten
- 2 cloves garlic, minced
- 1 tablespoon fresh parsley, chopped
- 1 teaspoon dried oregano
- 1/2 teaspoon sea salt
- 1/4 teaspoon black pepper
- 2 tablespoons olive oil
- 1 can (28 ounces) crushed tomatoes
- 1 teaspoon dried basil

Instructions:

1. In a large bowl, combine ground turkey, whole wheat breadcrumbs, grated Parmesan cheese, beaten egg, minced garlic, fresh parsley, dried oregano, sea salt, and black pepper. Mix well and form into meatballs.
2. Heat the olive oil in a large skillet over medium heat.
3. Add the meatballs and cook for 5-7 minutes, turning occasionally, until browned on all sides.
4. Add the crushed tomatoes and dried basil to the skillet. Stir to combine.
5. Reduce the heat and simmer for 20 minutes, until the meatballs are cooked through and the sauce has thickened.
6. Serve immediately.

Nutrition Info per Serving:

- Calories: 280
- Carbohydrates: 10g
- Protein: 28g
- Fat: 14g
- Fiber: 2g
- Sugar: 5g

Number of Servings: 4
Cooking Time: 30 minutes

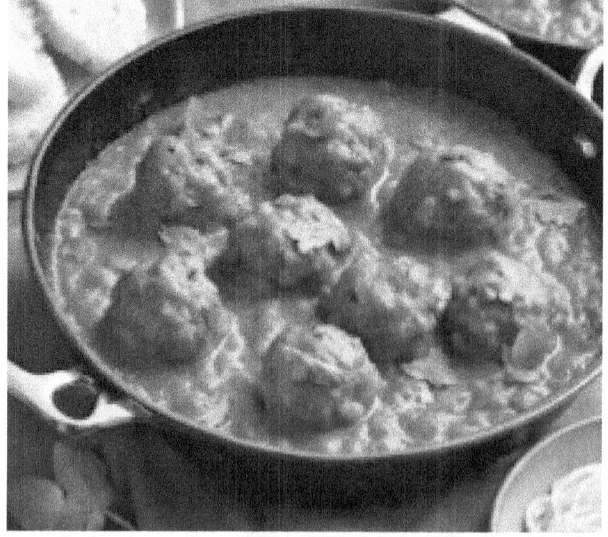

5. Turkey Chili

Ingredients:

- 1 tablespoon olive oil
- 1 onion, diced
- 2 cloves garlic, minced
- 1 red bell pepper, diced
- 1 green bell pepper, diced
- 1 pound ground turkey
- 2 tablespoons chili powder
- 1 teaspoon ground cumin
- 1 teaspoon paprika
- 1/2 teaspoon sea salt
- 1/4 teaspoon black pepper
- 1 can (14.5 ounces) diced tomatoes
- 1 can (15 ounces) kidney beans, drained and rinsed
- 1 cup low-sodium chicken broth
- 1/4 cup fresh cilantro, chopped

Instructions:

1. Heat the olive oil in a large pot over medium heat.
2. Add the onion, garlic, red bell pepper, and green bell pepper. Cook for 5-7 minutes, until softened.
3. Add the ground turkey and cook for another 5-7 minutes, until browned.
4. Stir in the chili powder, ground cumin, paprika, sea salt, and black pepper. Cook for 1 minute.
5. Add the diced tomatoes, kidney beans, and chicken broth. Bring to a boil, then reduce the heat and simmer for 20 minutes.
6. Stir in the fresh cilantro before serving.
7. Serve immediately.

Nutrition Info per Serving:

- Calories: 300
- Carbohydrates: 25g
- Protein: 30g
- Fat: 10g
- Fiber: 8g
- Sugar: 7g

Number of Servings: 4

Cooking Time: 40 minutes

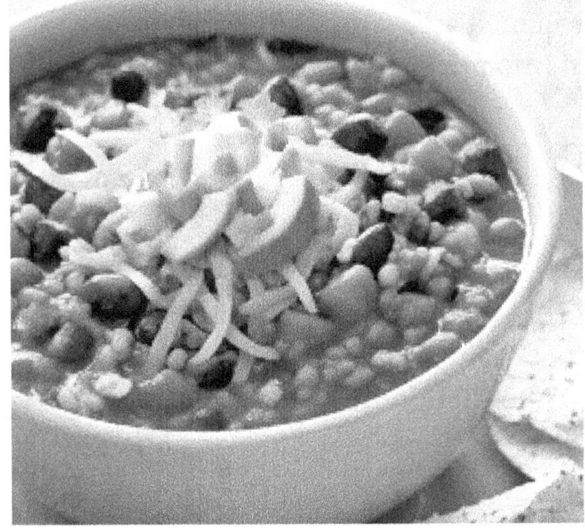

6. Chicken Lettuce Wraps

Ingredients:

- 1 pound ground chicken
- 1 tablespoon olive oil
- 1 onion, finely chopped
- 2 cloves garlic, minced
- 1 red bell pepper, diced
- 1/4 cup hoisin sauce
- 2 tablespoons soy sauce (low-sodium)
- 1 tablespoon rice vinegar
- 1 teaspoon fresh ginger, grated
- 1/4 teaspoon sea salt
- 1/4 teaspoon black pepper
- 1 cup water chestnuts, diced
- 1/4 cup green onions, chopped
- 1/4 cup fresh cilantro, chopped
- 1 head butter lettuce, leaves separated

Instructions:

1. Heat the olive oil in a large skillet over medium heat. Add the onion and cook for 2-3 minutes until softened.
2. Add the garlic and red bell pepper and cook for another 2 minutes.
3. Add the ground chicken and cook, breaking it up with a spoon, until fully cooked, about 5-7 minutes.
4. Stir in the hoisin sauce, soy sauce, rice vinegar, grated ginger, sea salt, and black pepper. Cook for another 2-3 minutes.
5. Add the water chestnuts and cook for 1-2 minutes until heated through.
6. Remove from heat and stir in the green onions and fresh cilantro.
7. Spoon the chicken mixture into the lettuce leaves.
8. Serve immediately.

Nutrition Info per Serving:

- Calories: 220
- Carbohydrates: 14g
- Protein: 24g
- Fat: 8g
- Fiber: 3g
- Sugar: 8g

Number of Servings: 4

Cooking Time: 20 minutes

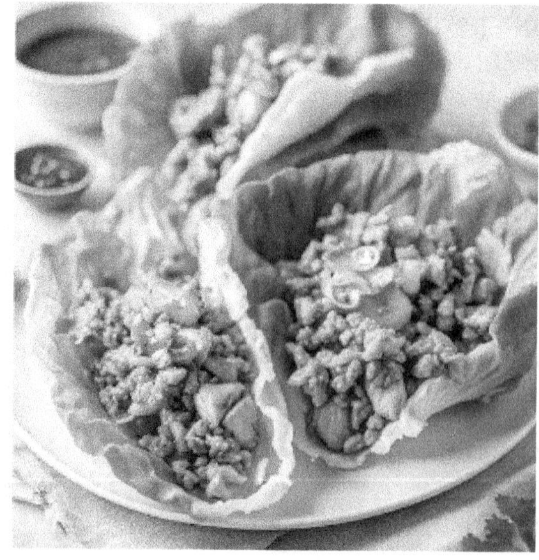

7. Mediterranean Stuffed Chicken

Ingredients:

- 4 boneless, skinless chicken breasts
- 1/2 cup sun-dried tomatoes, chopped
- 1/2 cup spinach, chopped
- 1/4 cup feta cheese, crumbled
- 1/4 cup Kalamata olives, chopped
- 2 cloves garlic, minced
- 1 tablespoon olive oil
- 1 teaspoon dried oregano
- 1/4 teaspoon sea salt
- 1/4 teaspoon black pepper

Instructions:

1. Preheat the oven to 375°F (190°C).
2. In a bowl, mix together sun-dried tomatoes, spinach, feta cheese, Kalamata olives, minced garlic, dried oregano, sea salt, and black pepper.
3. Cut a pocket into the side of each chicken breast.
4. Stuff the chicken breasts with the tomato mixture and secure with toothpicks.
5. Heat the olive oil in a large oven-safe skillet over medium-high heat.
6. Sear the chicken breasts for 2-3 minutes on each side until golden brown.
7. Transfer the skillet to the oven and bake for 20-25 minutes until the chicken is cooked through and the internal temperature reaches 165°F (74°C).
8. Serve immediately.

Nutrition Info per Serving:

- Calories: 300
- Carbohydrates: 6g
- Protein: 38g
- Fat: 14g
- Fiber: 2g
- Sugar: 3g

Number of Servings: 4
Cooking Time: 35 minutes

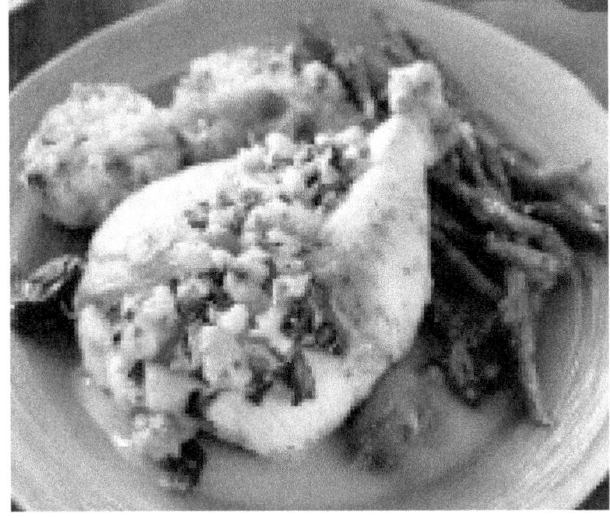

8. Chicken Cacciatore

Ingredients:

- 1 tablespoon olive oil
- 4 boneless, skinless chicken thighs
- 1 onion, diced
- 2 cloves garlic, minced
- 1 red bell pepper, sliced
- 1 yellow bell pepper, sliced
- 1 cup mushrooms, sliced
- 1 can (14.5 ounces) diced tomatoes
- 1/2 cup low-sodium chicken broth
- 1/2 cup dry white wine (optional)
- 1 teaspoon dried oregano
- 1 teaspoon dried basil
- 1/4 teaspoon sea salt
- 1/4 teaspoon black pepper
- 1/4 cup fresh parsley, chopped

Instructions:

1. Heat the olive oil in a large skillet over medium-high heat.
2. Add the chicken thighs and cook for 5-6 minutes on each side until browned. Remove from the skillet and set aside.
3. In the same skillet, add the onion, garlic, red bell pepper, yellow bell pepper, and mushrooms. Cook for 5-7 minutes until softened.
4. Stir in the diced tomatoes, chicken broth, white wine (if using), dried oregano, dried basil, sea salt, and black pepper.
5. Return the chicken to the skillet and bring to a simmer. Cover and cook for 25-30 minutes until the chicken is cooked through and the sauce has thickened.
6. Stir in the fresh parsley before serving.
7. Serve immediately.

Nutrition Info per Serving:

- Calories: 320
- Carbohydrates: 12g
- Protein: 30g
- Fat: 16g
- Fiber: 3g
- Sugar: 6g

Number of Servings: 4

Cooking Time: 45 minutes

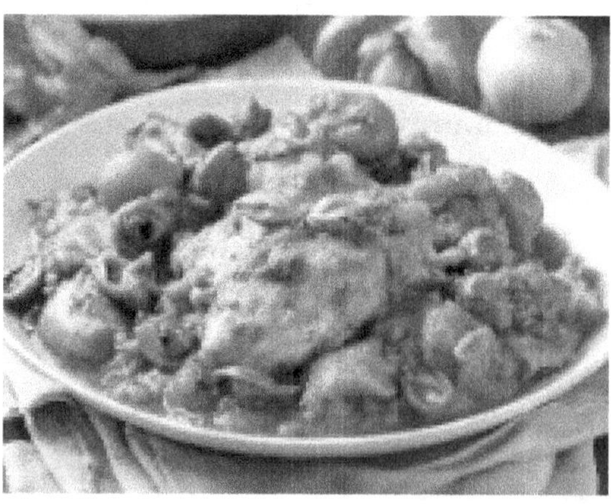

9. Turkey and Sweet Potato Skillet

Ingredients:
- 1 tablespoon olive oil
- 1 pound ground turkey
- 1 onion, diced
- 2 cloves garlic, minced
- 2 medium sweet potatoes, peeled and diced
- 1 red bell pepper, diced
- 1 teaspoon ground cumin
- 1 teaspoon paprika
- 1/4 teaspoon sea salt
- 1/4 teaspoon black pepper
- 1/4 cup fresh cilantro, chopped

Instructions:
1. Heat the olive oil in a large skillet over medium heat.
2. Add the ground turkey and cook for 5-7 minutes until browned. Remove from the skillet and set aside.
3. In the same skillet, add the onion, garlic, sweet potatoes, and red bell pepper. Cook for 8-10 minutes until the sweet potatoes are tender.
4. Stir in the ground cumin, paprika, sea salt, and black pepper. Cook for another 2-3 minutes.
5. Return the ground turkey to the skillet and stir to combine. Cook for another 2-3 minutes until heated through.
6. Stir in the fresh cilantro before serving.
7. Serve immediately.

Nutrition Info per Serving:
- Calories: 320
- Carbohydrates: 25g
- Protein: 28g
- Fat: 12g
- Fiber: 6g
- Sugar: 8g

Number of Servings: 4
Cooking Time: 30 minutes

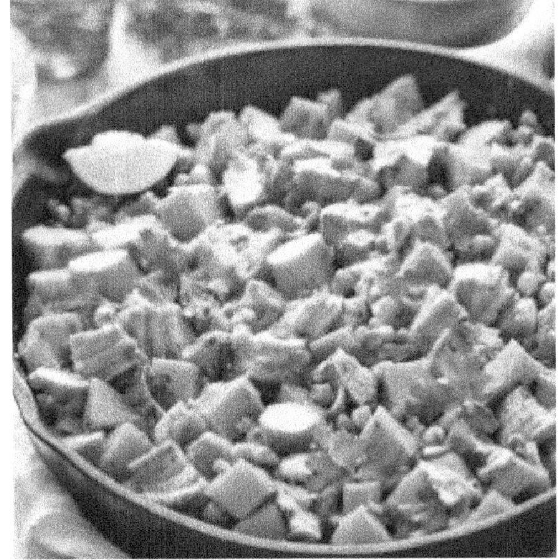

10. Chicken Curry with Coconut Milk

Ingredients:

- 1 tablespoon olive oil
- 1 onion, diced
- 2 cloves garlic, minced
- 1 tablespoon fresh ginger, grated
- 1 pound boneless, skinless chicken breasts, cut into bite-sized pieces
- 2 tablespoons curry powder
- 1 teaspoon ground turmeric
- 1 can (14.5 ounces) coconut milk
- 1 cup low-sodium chicken broth
- 1 red bell pepper, sliced
- 1 cup snap peas
- 1/4 teaspoon sea salt
- 1/4 teaspoon black pepper
- 1/4 cup fresh cilantro, chopped

Instructions:

1. Heat the olive oil in a large pot over medium heat.
2. Add the onion, garlic, and ginger. Cook for 5-7 minutes until softened.
3. Add the chicken pieces and cook for another 5 minutes until lightly browned.
4. Stir in the curry powder and ground turmeric. Cook for 1 minute until fragrant.
5. Pour in the coconut milk and chicken broth. Bring to a simmer.
6. Add the red bell pepper and snap peas. Cook for 10-15 minutes until the chicken is cooked through and the vegetables are tender.
7. Stir in the sea salt, black pepper, and fresh cilantro.
8. Serve immediately.

Nutrition Info per Serving:

- Calories: 350
- Carbohydrates: 12g
- Protein: 32g
- Fat: 20g
- Fiber: 4g
- Sugar: 4g

Number of Servings: 4

Cooking Time: 35 minutes

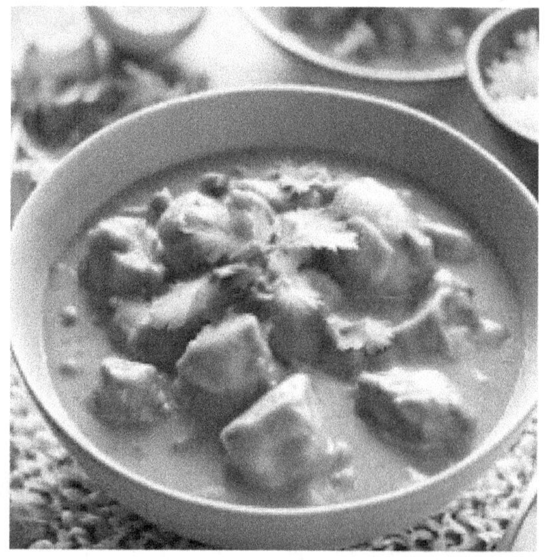

11. Turkey Breast with Apple Salsa

Ingredients:

- 1 pound turkey breast, skinless
- 2 tablespoons olive oil
- 1 teaspoon dried thyme
- 1/4 teaspoon sea salt
- 1/4 teaspoon black pepper
- 2 apples, diced
- 1/4 red onion, finely chopped
- 1/4 cup fresh cilantro, chopped
- 1 tablespoon lime juice
- 1 teaspoon honey

Instructions:

1. Preheat the oven to 375°F (190°C).
2. Rub the turkey breast with olive oil, dried thyme, sea salt, and black pepper.
3. Place the turkey breast in a baking dish and bake for 25-30 minutes, or until the internal temperature reaches 165°F (74°C).
4. While the turkey is baking, prepare the apple salsa by combining the diced apples, red onion, cilantro, lime juice, and honey in a bowl.
5. Once the turkey is done, let it rest for 5 minutes before slicing.
6. Serve the turkey breast topped with apple salsa.

Nutrition Info per Serving:

- Calories: 280
- Carbohydrates: 12g
- Protein: 30g
- Fat: 12g
- Fiber: 3g
- Sugar: 8g

Number of Servings: 4
Cooking Time: 35 minutes

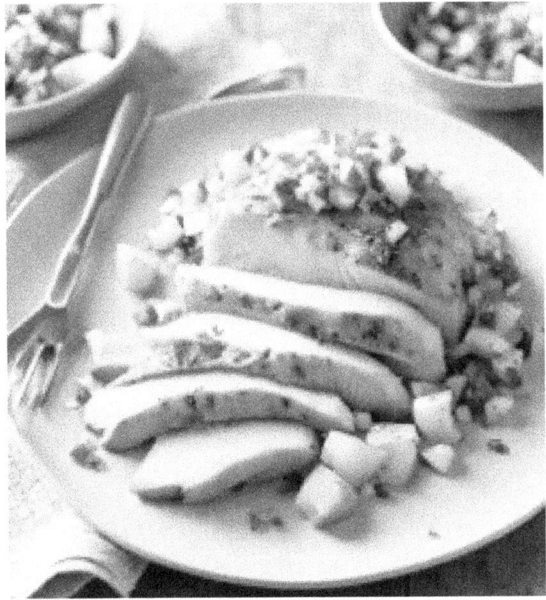

12. Slow Cooker Chicken Stew

Ingredients:

- 1 pound boneless, skinless chicken thighs, cut into chunks
- 2 cups low-sodium chicken broth
- 1 onion, diced
- 3 carrots, sliced
- 2 celery stalks, sliced
- 2 potatoes, diced
- 2 cloves garlic, minced
- 1 teaspoon dried thyme
- 1 teaspoon dried rosemary
- 1/2 teaspoon sea salt
- 1/4 teaspoon black pepper
- 1 cup frozen peas

Instructions:

1. Place the chicken chunks, chicken broth, onion, carrots, celery, potatoes, garlic, dried thyme, dried rosemary, sea salt, and black pepper in a slow cooker.
2. Cover and cook on low for 6-7 hours or on high for 3-4 hours.
3. About 30 minutes before serving, add the frozen peas.
4. Serve warm.

Nutrition Info per Serving:

- Calories: 300
- Carbohydrates: 28g
- Protein: 25g
- Fat: 10g
- Fiber: 5g
- Sugar: 7g

Number of Servings: 4
Cooking Time: 6-7 hours

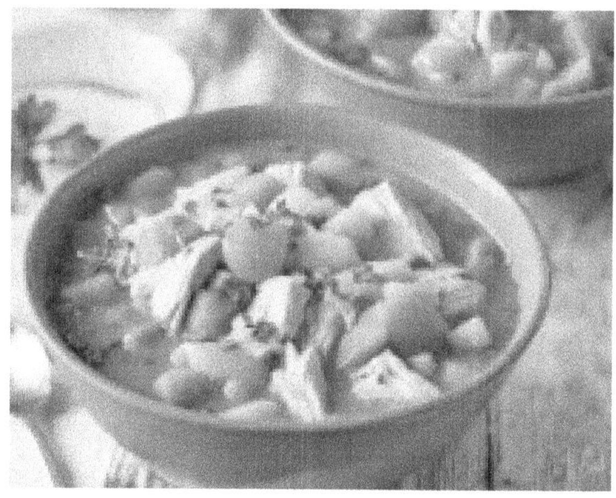

13. Balsamic Glazed Chicken

Ingredients:

- 4 boneless, skinless chicken breasts
- 2 tablespoons olive oil
- 1/4 cup balsamic vinegar
- 2 tablespoons honey
- 1 teaspoon dried basil
- 1/4 teaspoon sea salt
- 1/4 teaspoon black pepper
- 1 cup cherry tomatoes, halved
- 1/4 cup fresh basil, chopped

Instructions:

1. Heat the olive oil in a large skillet over medium heat.
2. Add the chicken breasts and cook for 5-6 minutes on each side until golden brown and cooked through.
3. Remove the chicken from the skillet and set aside.
4. In the same skillet, add balsamic vinegar, honey, dried basil, sea salt, and black pepper. Bring to a simmer and cook for 2-3 minutes until the sauce thickens.
5. Return the chicken to the skillet and coat with the balsamic glaze.
6. Add the cherry tomatoes and cook for another 2 minutes.
7. Serve the chicken topped with fresh basil.

Nutrition Info per Serving:

- Calories: 280
- Carbohydrates: 16g
- Protein: 30g
- Fat: 12g
- Fiber: 2g
- Sugar: 14g

Number of Servings: 4
Cooking Time: 20 minutes

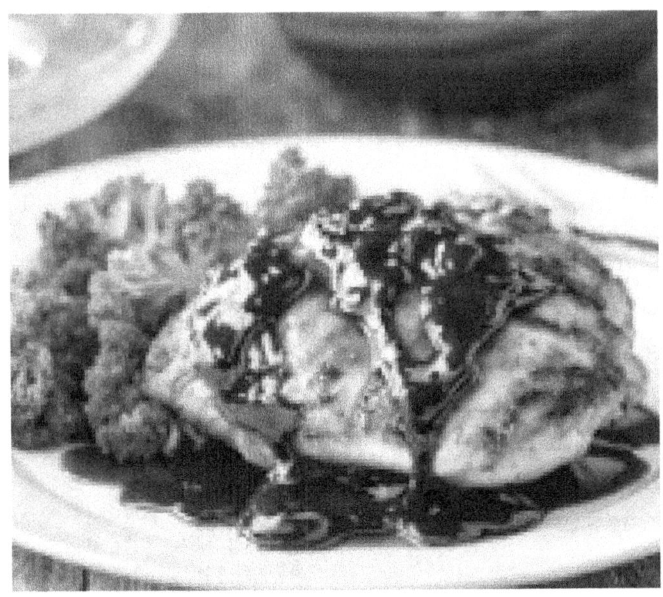

14. Asian Chicken Noodle Soup

Ingredients:

- 1 tablespoon olive oil
- 1 pound boneless, skinless chicken thighs, cut into bite-sized pieces
- 1 onion, diced
- 2 cloves garlic, minced
- 1 tablespoon fresh ginger, grated
- 8 cups low-sodium chicken broth
- 1 cup carrots, julienned
- 1 cup snow peas, trimmed
- 1 red bell pepper, sliced
- 4 ounces rice noodles
- 1/4 cup low-sodium soy sauce
- 1 tablespoon sesame oil
- 1/4 cup fresh cilantro, chopped

Instructions:

1. Heat the olive oil in a large pot over medium heat.
2. Add the chicken and cook for 5-7 minutes until browned.
3. Add the onion, garlic, and ginger. Cook for another 3-4 minutes until fragrant.
4. Pour in the chicken broth and bring to a boil. Reduce heat and simmer for 10 minutes.
5. Add the carrots, snow peas, and red bell pepper. Cook for another 5 minutes.
6. Stir in the rice noodles, soy sauce, and sesame oil. Cook for another 3-4 minutes until the noodles are tender.
7. Stir in the fresh cilantro before serving.
8. Serve warm.

Nutrition Info per Serving:

- Calories: 280
- Carbohydrates: 22g
- Protein: 28g
- Fat: 10g
- Fiber: 3g
- Sugar: 6g

Number of Servings: 4
Cooking Time: 30 minutes

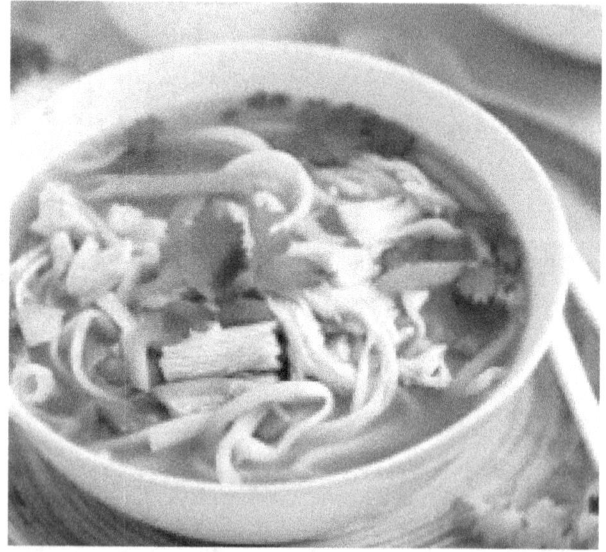

15. Chicken Piccata

Ingredients:

- 4 boneless, skinless chicken breasts
- 1/4 cup whole wheat flour
- 2 tablespoons olive oil
- 1/2 cup low-sodium chicken broth
- 1/4 cup lemon juice
- 2 tablespoons capers, drained
- 1/4 teaspoon sea salt
- 1/4 teaspoon black pepper
- 1/4 cup fresh parsley, chopped

Instructions:

1. Lightly coat the chicken breasts with whole wheat flour.
2. Heat the olive oil in a large skillet over medium heat.
3. Add the chicken breasts and cook for 4-5 minutes on each side until golden brown and cooked through. Remove from the skillet and set aside.
4. In the same skillet, add the chicken broth, lemon juice, capers, sea salt, and black pepper. Bring to a simmer and cook for 2-3 minutes until the sauce thickens.
5. Return the chicken to the skillet and coat with the sauce.
6. Serve the chicken topped with fresh parsley.

Nutrition Info per Serving:

- Calories: 250
- Carbohydrates: 10g
- Protein: 30g
- Fat: 10g
- Fiber: 1g
- Sugar: 1g

Number of Servings: 4
Cooking Time: 20 minutes

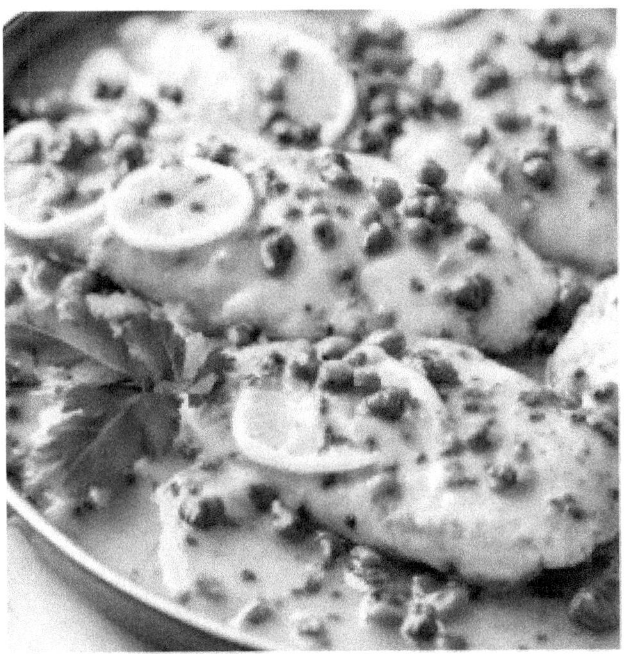

16. Turkey Stuffed Peppers

Ingredients:

- 4 large bell peppers
- 1 pound ground turkey
- 1 tablespoon olive oil
- 1 onion, diced
- 2 cloves garlic, minced
- 1 cup cooked quinoa
- 1 can (14.5 ounces) diced tomatoes
- 1 teaspoon dried oregano
- 1/4 teaspoon sea salt
- 1/4 teaspoon black pepper
- 1/2 cup shredded mozzarella cheese
- 1/4 cup fresh parsley, chopped

Instructions:

1. Preheat the oven to 375°F (190°C).
2. Cut the tops off the bell peppers and remove the seeds and membranes. Place the peppers in a baking dish.
3. Heat the olive oil in a large skillet over medium heat.
4. Add the ground turkey, onion, and garlic. Cook for 5-7 minutes until the turkey is browned and the onion is softened.
5. Stir in the cooked quinoa, diced tomatoes, dried oregano, sea salt, and black pepper. Cook for another 3-4 minutes.
6. Stuff the bell peppers with the turkey mixture and top with shredded mozzarella cheese.
7. Cover the baking dish with foil and bake for 25 minutes. Remove the foil and bake for an additional 10 minutes until the cheese is melted and bubbly.
8. Sprinkle with fresh parsley before serving.
9. Serve immediately.

Nutrition Info per Serving:

- Calories: 320
- Carbohydrates: 22g
- Protein: 30g
- Fat: 14g
- Fiber: 5g
- Sugar: 8g

Number of Servings: 4

Cooking Time: 45 minutes

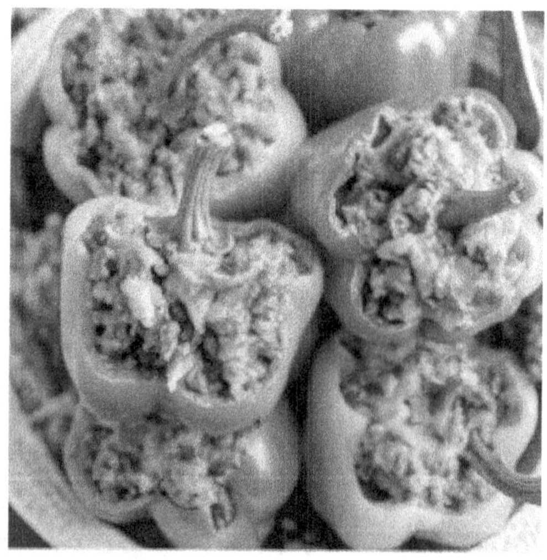

17. Chicken Ratatouille

Ingredients:

- 1 pound boneless, skinless chicken breasts, cut into bite-sized pieces
- 2 tablespoons olive oil
- 1 onion, diced
- 2 cloves garlic, minced
- 1 eggplant, diced
- 1 zucchini, sliced
- 1 yellow squash, sliced
- 1 red bell pepper, diced
- 1 can (14.5 ounces) diced tomatoes
- 1 teaspoon dried thyme
- 1 teaspoon dried basil
- 1/4 teaspoon sea salt
- 1/4 teaspoon black pepper
- 1/4 cup fresh basil, chopped

Instructions:

1. Heat 1 tablespoon of olive oil in a large skillet over medium heat.
2. Add the chicken pieces and cook for 5-7 minutes until browned and cooked through. Remove from the skillet and set aside.
3. In the same skillet, heat the remaining tablespoon of olive oil. Add the onion and garlic, and cook for 2-3 minutes until softened.
4. Add the eggplant, zucchini, yellow squash, and red bell pepper. Cook for 5-7 minutes until the vegetables are tender.
5. Stir in the diced tomatoes, dried thyme, dried basil, sea salt, and black pepper. Cook for another 5 minutes.
6. Return the chicken to the skillet and cook for 2-3 minutes until heated through.
7. Remove from heat and stir in the fresh basil.
8. Serve immediately.

Nutrition Info per Serving:

- Calories: 250
- Carbohydrates: 15g
- Protein: 28g
- Fat: 10g
- Fiber: 5g
- Sugar: 8g

Number of Servings: 4

Cooking Time: 30 minutes

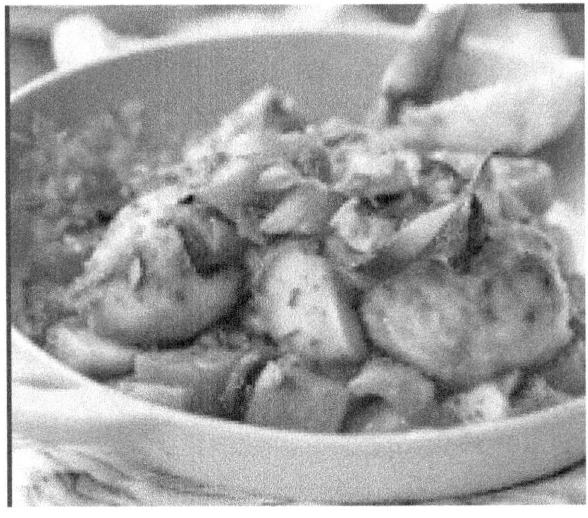

18. Moroccan Chicken Tagine
Ingredients:

- 1 pound boneless, skinless chicken thighs, cut into bite-sized pieces
- 2 tablespoons olive oil
- 1 onion, diced
- 2 cloves garlic, minced
- 1 teaspoon ground cumin
- 1 teaspoon ground cinnamon
- 1 teaspoon ground ginger
- 1/2 teaspoon turmeric
- 1/4 teaspoon sea salt
- 1/4 teaspoon black pepper
- 1 cup low-sodium chicken broth
- 1 cup diced tomatoes
- 1/2 cup dried apricots, chopped
- 1/4 cup green olives, pitted and sliced
- 1/4 cup fresh cilantro, chopped

Instructions:

1. Heat 1 tablespoon of olive oil in a large pot or tagine over medium heat.
2. Add the chicken pieces and cook for 5-7 minutes until browned. Remove from the pot and set aside.
3. In the same pot, heat the remaining tablespoon of olive oil. Add the onion and garlic, and cook for 2-3 minutes until softened.
4. Stir in the ground cumin, ground cinnamon, ground ginger, turmeric, sea salt, and black pepper. Cook for 1 minute until fragrant.
5. Add the chicken broth, diced tomatoes, dried apricots, and green olives. Bring to a simmer.
6. Return the chicken to the pot and cook for 20-25 minutes until the chicken is cooked through and the flavors have melded together.
7. Remove from heat and stir in the fresh cilantro.
8. Serve immediately.

Nutrition Info per Serving:

- Calories: 320
- Carbohydrates: 20g
- Protein: 28g
- Fat: 14g
- Fiber: 4g
- Sugar: 10g

Number of Servings: 4
Cooking Time: 35 minutes

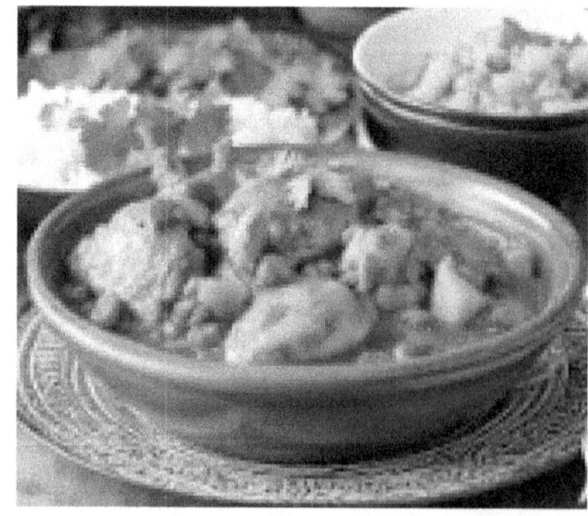

19. Buffalo Chicken Salad

Ingredients:

- 1 pound boneless, skinless chicken breasts
- 2 tablespoons olive oil
- 1/4 cup hot sauce (such as Frank's RedHot)
- 6 cups mixed greens (spinach, arugula, lettuce)
- 1 cup cherry tomatoes, halved
- 1/2 cucumber, sliced
- 1/4 red onion, thinly sliced
- 1/4 cup blue cheese crumbles (optional)
- 1/4 cup Greek yogurt
- 1 tablespoon lemon juice
- 1 teaspoon honey

Instructions:

1. Preheat the grill to medium-high heat.
2. In a small bowl, mix together 1 tablespoon of olive oil and the hot sauce.
3. Brush the mixture over the chicken breasts.
4. Grill the chicken for 6-7 minutes on each side until cooked through. Remove from the grill and let it rest for 5 minutes before slicing.
5. In a large bowl, combine the mixed greens, cherry tomatoes, cucumber, and red onion.
6. Top the salad with the sliced grilled chicken and blue cheese crumbles (if using).
7. In a small bowl, mix together the Greek yogurt, lemon juice, honey, and remaining tablespoon of olive oil.
8. Drizzle the dressing over the salad.
9. Serve immediately.

Nutrition Info per Serving:

- Calories: 300
- Carbohydrates: 10g
- Protein: 34g
- Fat: 14g
- Fiber: 3g
- Sugar: 5g

Number of Servings: 4
Cooking Time: 20 minutes

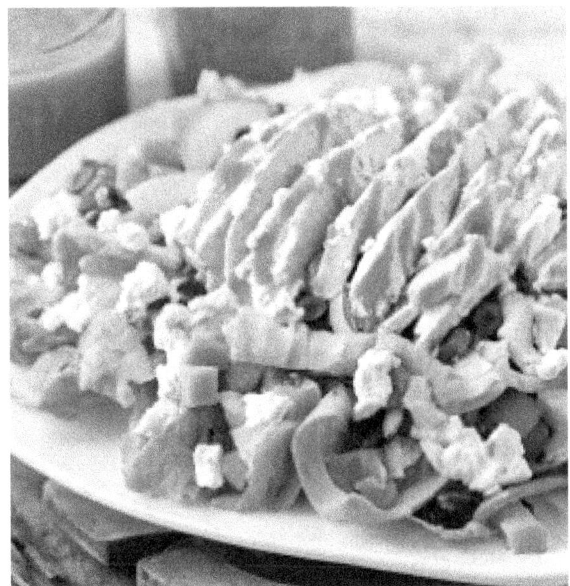

20. Chicken Paillard

Ingredients:

- 4 boneless, skinless chicken breasts
- 2 tablespoons olive oil
- 1 lemon, juiced
- 1 teaspoon dried thyme
- 1/4 teaspoon sea salt
- 1/4 teaspoon black pepper
- 4 cups mixed greens (spinach, arugula, lettuce)
- 1/2 cup cherry tomatoes, halved
- 1/4 cup red onion, thinly sliced
- 1/4 cup fresh parsley, chopped

Instructions:

1. Preheat the grill to medium-high heat.
2. Pound the chicken breasts to an even thickness.
3. In a small bowl, mix together 1 tablespoon of olive oil, lemon juice, dried thyme, sea salt, and black pepper.
4. Brush the mixture over the chicken breasts.
5. Grill the chicken for 4-5 minutes on each side until cooked through.
6. In a large bowl, combine the mixed greens, cherry tomatoes, red onion, and fresh parsley.
7. Slice the grilled chicken and place on top of the salad.
8. Drizzle the remaining tablespoon of olive oil over the salad.
9. Serve immediately.

Nutrition Info per Serving:

- Calories: 270
- Carbohydrates: 8g
- Protein: 34g
- Fat: 12g
- Fiber: 3g
- Sugar: 4g

Number of Servings: 4
Cooking Time: 20 minutes

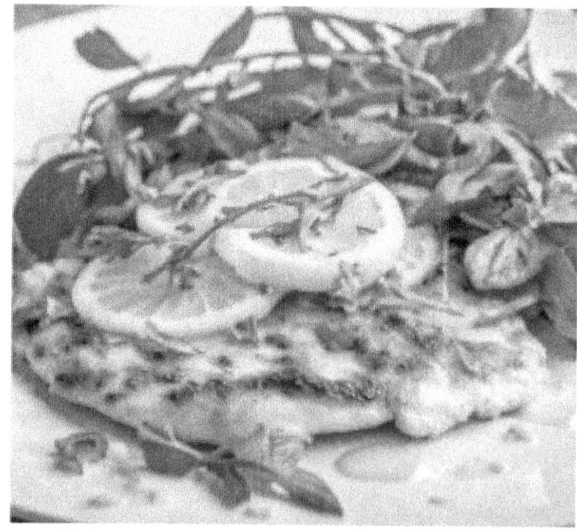

21. Turkey Soup with Kale

Ingredients:

- 1 tablespoon olive oil
- 1 pound ground turkey
- 1 onion, diced
- 2 cloves garlic, minced
- 2 carrots, sliced
- 2 celery stalks, sliced
- 6 cups low-sodium chicken broth
- 1 can (14.5 ounces) diced tomatoes
- 1 teaspoon dried thyme
- 1/2 teaspoon dried rosemary
- 1/4 teaspoon sea salt
- 1/4 teaspoon black pepper
- 2 cups chopped kale

Instructions:

1. Heat the olive oil in a large pot over medium heat.
2. Add the ground turkey and cook for 5-7 minutes until browned. Remove from the pot and set aside.
3. In the same pot, add the onion, garlic, carrots, and celery. Cook for 5-7 minutes until softened.
4. Stir in the chicken broth, diced tomatoes, dried thyme, dried rosemary, sea salt, and black pepper. Bring to a simmer.
5. Return the turkey to the pot and cook for 10 minutes.
6. Add the chopped kale and cook for another 5 minutes until the kale is tender.
7. Serve warm.

Nutrition Info per Serving:

- Calories: 280
- Carbohydrates: 14g
- Protein: 30g
- Fat: 12g
- Fiber: 4g
- Sugar: 6g

Number of Servings: 4
Cooking Time: 30 minutes

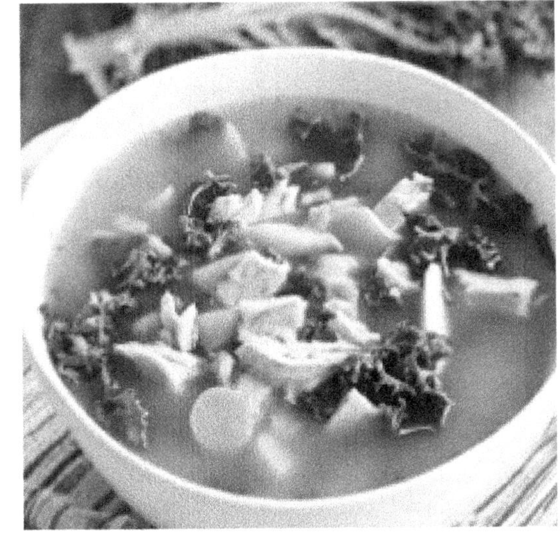

22. Sesame Ginger Chicken

Ingredients:

- 1 pound boneless, skinless chicken breasts, cut into strips
- 2 tablespoons olive oil
- 2 tablespoons low-sodium soy sauce
- 1 tablespoon sesame oil
- 1 tablespoon honey
- 1 tablespoon fresh ginger, grated
- 2 cloves garlic, minced
- 1 tablespoon sesame seeds
- 2 green onions, chopped

Instructions:

1. In a small bowl, mix together soy sauce, sesame oil, honey, grated ginger, and minced garlic.
2. Heat olive oil in a large skillet over medium heat.
3. Add the chicken strips and cook for 5-7 minutes, until browned and cooked through.
4. Pour the soy sauce mixture over the chicken and cook for an additional 2-3 minutes, until the sauce thickens.
5. Sprinkle with sesame seeds and green onions before serving.
6. Serve immediately.

Nutrition Info per Serving:

- Calories: 280
- Carbohydrates: 8g
- Protein: 32g
- Fat: 14g
- Fiber: 1g
- Sugar: 6g

Number of Servings: 4
Cooking Time: 20 minutes

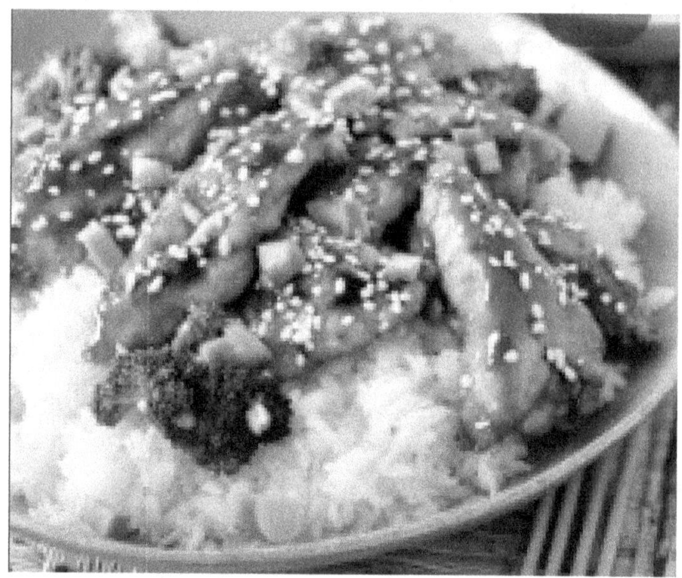

23. Barbecue Chicken Breast

Ingredients:

- 4 boneless, skinless chicken breasts
- 1/2 cup barbecue sauce (low-sugar)
- 1 tablespoon olive oil
- 1 teaspoon smoked paprika
- 1/4 teaspoon sea salt
- 1/4 teaspoon black pepper

Instructions:

1. Preheat the grill to medium-high heat.
2. In a small bowl, mix together the barbecue sauce, olive oil, smoked paprika, sea salt, and black pepper.
3. Brush the chicken breasts with the barbecue sauce mixture.
4. Grill the chicken for 6-7 minutes on each side, until cooked through and the internal temperature reaches 165°F (74°C).
5. Let the chicken rest for 5 minutes before serving.
6. Serve immediately.

Nutrition Info per Serving:

- Calories: 250
- Carbohydrates: 10g
- Protein: 32g
- Fat: 10g
- Fiber: 1g
- Sugar: 8g

Number of Servings: 4
Cooking Time: 20 minutes

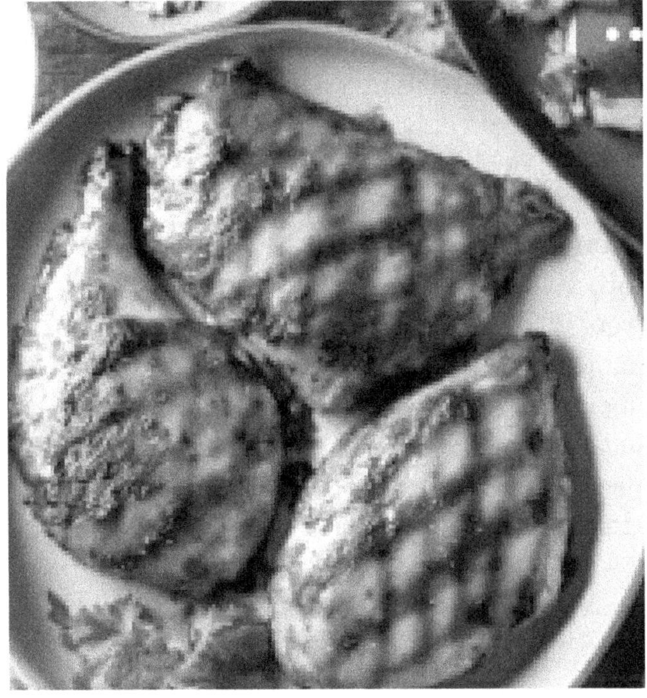

24. Chicken Bruschetta

Ingredients:

- 4 boneless, skinless chicken breasts
- 2 tablespoons olive oil
- 1 teaspoon dried basil
- 1/4 teaspoon sea salt
- 1/4 teaspoon black pepper
- 4 Roma tomatoes, diced
- 2 cloves garlic, minced
- 1/4 cup fresh basil, chopped
- 1 tablespoon balsamic vinegar

Instructions:

1. Preheat the oven to 375°F (190°C).
2. In a small bowl, mix together 1 tablespoon of olive oil, dried basil, sea salt, and black pepper.
3. Brush the mixture over the chicken breasts.
4. Heat the remaining tablespoon of olive oil in a large skillet over medium heat.
5. Add the chicken breasts and cook for 2-3 minutes on each side until browned.
6. Transfer the chicken to a baking dish and bake for 20-25 minutes, until the internal temperature reaches 165°F (74°C).
7. While the chicken is baking, mix together the diced tomatoes, minced garlic, fresh basil, and balsamic vinegar in a bowl.
8. Top the baked chicken with the tomato mixture before serving.
9. Serve immediately.

Nutrition Info per Serving:

- Calories: 280
- Carbohydrates: 8g
- Protein: 32g
- Fat: 14g
- Fiber: 2g
- Sugar: 5g

Number of Servings: 4
Cooking Time: 30 minutes

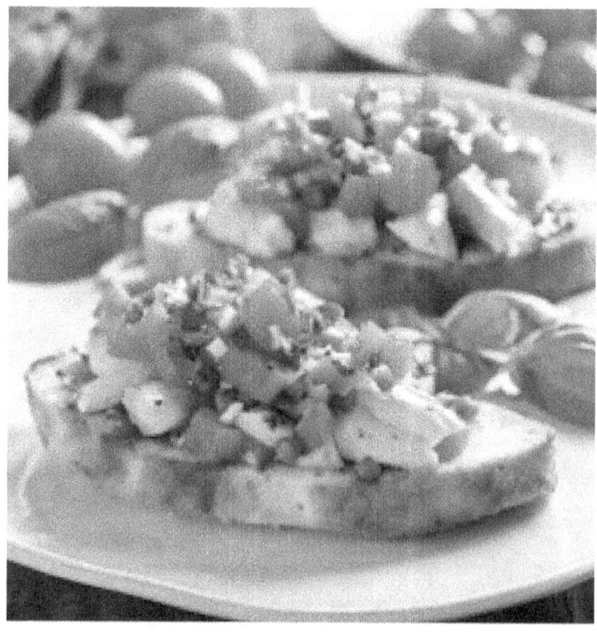

25. Herb Roasted Turkey

Ingredients:

- 1 whole turkey breast (about 4 pounds)
- 2 tablespoons olive oil
- 1 tablespoon fresh rosemary, chopped
- 1 tablespoon fresh thyme, chopped
- 1 tablespoon fresh sage, chopped
- 1/4 teaspoon sea salt
- 1/4 teaspoon black pepper
- 1 lemon, sliced
- 4 cloves garlic, minced

Instructions:

1. Preheat the oven to 375°F (190°C).
2. In a small bowl, mix together olive oil, chopped rosemary, thyme, sage, minced garlic, sea salt, and black pepper.
3. Rub the mixture all over the turkey breast, including under the skin.
4. Place the lemon slices under the skin and in the cavity of the turkey breast.
5. Place the turkey breast in a roasting pan.
6. Roast for 1 hour and 30 minutes, or until the internal temperature reaches 165°F (74°C).
7. Let the turkey rest for 10 minutes before carving.
8. Serve immediately.

Nutrition Info per Serving:

- Calories: 300
- Carbohydrates: 2g
- Protein: 40g
- Fat: 14g
- Fiber: 1g
- Sugar: 0g

Number of Servings: 8
Cooking Time: 1 hour and 40 minutes

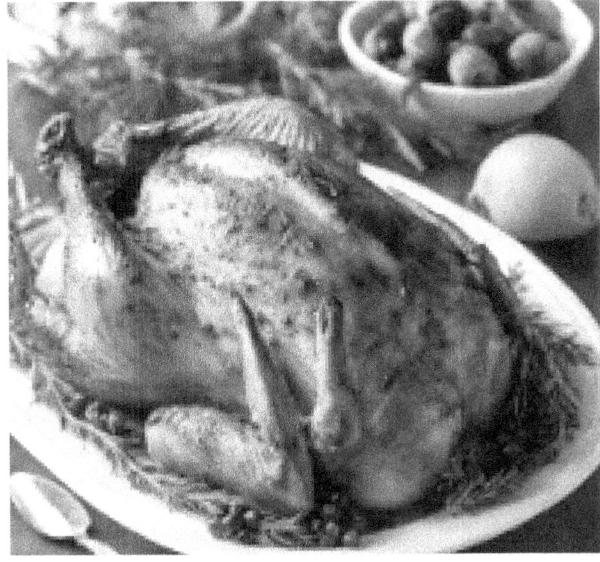

Soup & Stew recipes

1. Lentil Soup

Ingredients:

- 2 tablespoons olive oil
- 1 onion, diced
- 2 cloves garlic, minced
- 2 carrots, sliced
- 2 celery stalks, sliced
- 1 cup dried lentils, rinsed
- 6 cups low-sodium vegetable broth
- 1 can (14.5 ounces) diced tomatoes
- 1 teaspoon dried thyme
- 1 teaspoon ground cumin
- 1/4 teaspoon sea salt
- 1/4 teaspoon black pepper
- 1 bay leaf
- 2 cups chopped spinach

Instructions:

1. Heat the olive oil in a large pot over medium heat.
2. Add the onion, garlic, carrots, and celery. Cook for 5-7 minutes until softened.
3. Add the lentils, vegetable broth, diced tomatoes, dried thyme, ground cumin, sea salt, black pepper, and bay leaf.
4. Bring to a boil, then reduce heat and simmer for 30-35 minutes until the lentils are tender.
5. Stir in the chopped spinach and cook for an additional 5 minutes.
6. Remove the bay leaf before serving.
7. Serve warm.

Nutrition Info per Serving:

- Calories: 200
- Carbohydrates: 30g
- Protein: 10g
- Fat: 6g
- Fiber: 10g
- Sugar: 6g

Number of Servings: 6

Cooking Time: 45 minutes

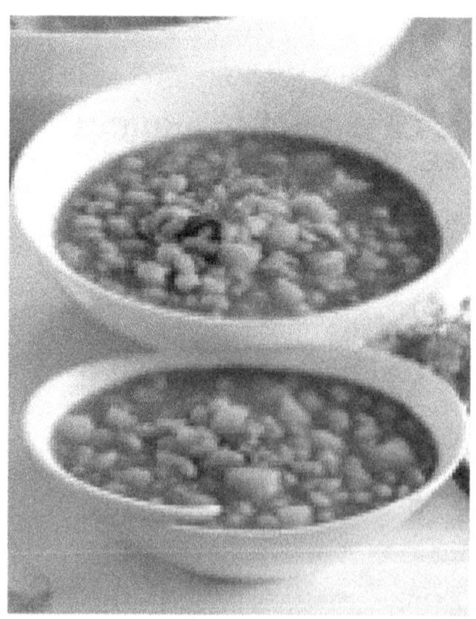

2. Carrot and Ginger Soup

Ingredients:

- 2 tablespoons olive oil
- 1 onion, diced
- 4 cups carrots, peeled and sliced
- 2 cloves garlic, minced
- 1 tablespoon fresh ginger, grated
- 6 cups low-sodium vegetable broth
- 1/4 teaspoon sea salt
- 1/4 teaspoon black pepper
- 1/4 cup coconut milk (optional)
- Fresh cilantro, chopped (for garnish)

Instructions:

1. Heat the olive oil in a large pot over medium heat.
2. Add the onion and cook for 5 minutes until softened.
3. Add the carrots, garlic, and ginger. Cook for another 5 minutes.
4. Pour in the vegetable broth and bring to a boil. Reduce heat and simmer for 20-25 minutes until the carrots are tender.
5. Use an immersion blender to puree the soup until smooth (or carefully transfer to a blender in batches).
6. Stir in the coconut milk (if using) and season with sea salt and black pepper.
7. Garnish with fresh cilantro before serving.
8. Serve warm.

Nutrition Info per Serving:

- Calories: 160
- Carbohydrates: 22g
- Protein: 3g
- Fat: 7g
- Fiber: 5g
- Sugar: 10g

Number of Servings: 6
Cooking Time: 35 minutes

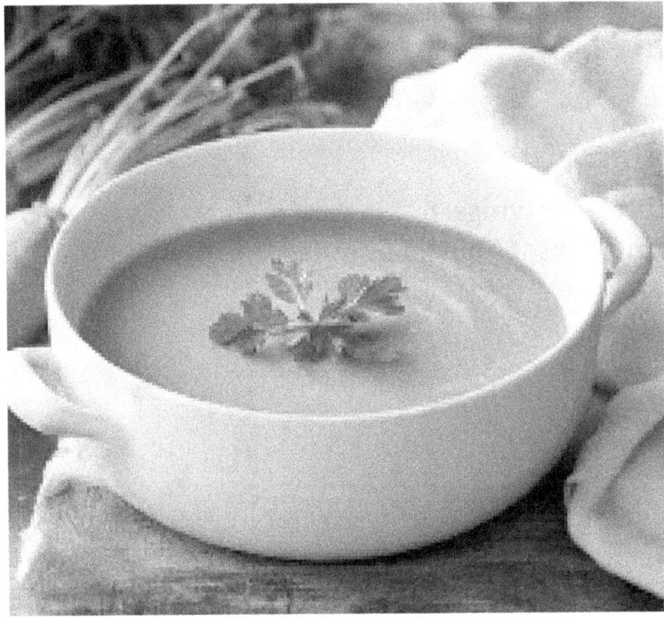

3. Split Pea Soup
Ingredients:
- 2 tablespoons olive oil
- 1 onion, diced
- 2 cloves garlic, minced
- 2 carrots, sliced
- 2 celery stalks, sliced
- 2 cups dried split peas, rinsed
- 6 cups low-sodium vegetable broth
- 1 bay leaf
- 1 teaspoon dried thyme
- 1/4 teaspoon sea salt
- 1/4 teaspoon black pepper

Instructions:
1. Heat the olive oil in a large pot over medium heat.
2. Add the onion, garlic, carrots, and celery. Cook for 5-7 minutes until softened.
3. Add the split peas, vegetable broth, bay leaf, dried thyme, sea salt, and black pepper.
4. Bring to a boil, then reduce heat and simmer for 1 hour, stirring occasionally, until the peas are tender and the soup has thickened.
5. Remove the bay leaf before serving.
6. Serve warm.

Nutrition Info per Serving:
- Calories: 220
- Carbohydrates: 36g
- Protein: 14g
- Fat: 5g
- Fiber: 12g
- Sugar: 6g

Number of Servings: 6
Cooking Time: 1 hour 15 minutes

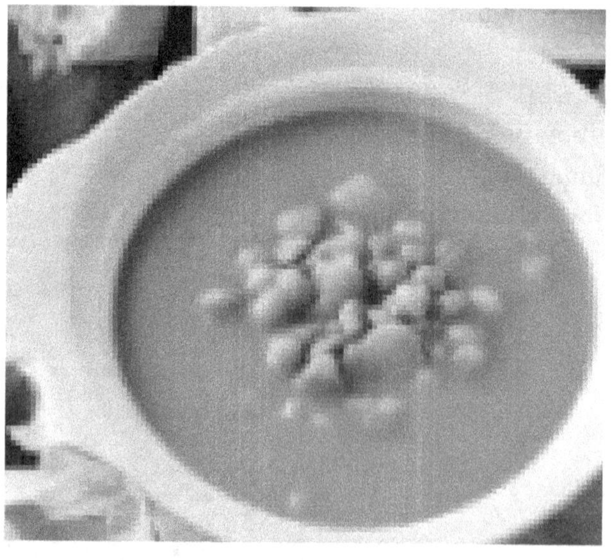

4. Beef Barley Soup

Ingredients:

- 1 pound beef stew meat, cut into bite-sized pieces
- 2 tablespoons olive oil
- 1 onion, diced
- 2 cloves garlic, minced
- 2 carrots, sliced
- 2 celery stalks, sliced
- 1 cup pearl barley
- 6 cups low-sodium beef broth
- 1 can (14.5 ounces) diced tomatoes
- 1 teaspoon dried thyme
- 1/4 teaspoon sea salt
- 1/4 teaspoon black pepper
- 2 cups chopped spinach

Instructions:

1. Heat 1 tablespoon of olive oil in a large pot over medium-high heat. Add the beef and cook until browned on all sides. Remove from the pot and set aside.
2. In the same pot, heat the remaining tablespoon of olive oil. Add the onion, garlic, carrots, and celery. Cook for 5-7 minutes until softened.
3. Stir in the pearl barley and cook for 1-2 minutes.
4. Add the beef broth, diced tomatoes, dried thyme, sea salt, and black pepper. Bring to a boil, then reduce heat and simmer for 45 minutes.
5. Return the beef to the pot and simmer for another 15 minutes, until the beef is tender and the barley is cooked.
6. Stir in the chopped spinach and cook for an additional 5 minutes.
7. Serve warm.

Nutrition Info per Serving:

- Calories: 300
- Carbohydrates: 30g
- Protein: 20g
- Fat: 10g
- Fiber: 8g
- Sugar: 7g

Number of Servings: 6
Cooking Time: 1 hour 15 minutes

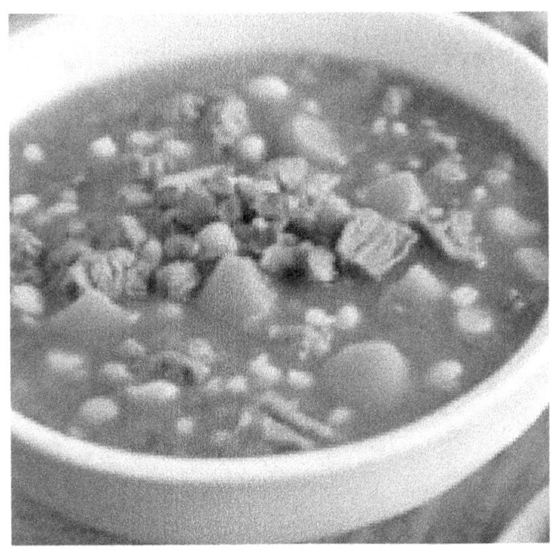

5. Tomato Basil Soup

Ingredients:

- 2 tablespoons olive oil
- 1 onion, diced
- 3 cloves garlic, minced
- 2 cans (28 ounces each) whole peeled tomatoes
- 4 cups low-sodium vegetable broth
- 1 teaspoon dried oregano
- 1/4 teaspoon sea salt
- 1/4 teaspoon black pepper
- 1/2 cup fresh basil, chopped
- 1/4 cup coconut milk (optional)

Instructions:

1. Heat the olive oil in a large pot over medium heat.
2. Add the onion and garlic, and cook for 5-7 minutes until softened.
3. Add the tomatoes, vegetable broth, dried oregano, sea salt, and black pepper. Bring to a boil, then reduce heat and simmer for 20-25 minutes.
4. Use an immersion blender to puree the soup until smooth (or carefully transfer to a blender in batches).
5. Stir in the fresh basil and coconut milk (if using).
6. Serve warm.

Nutrition Info per Serving:

- Calories: 180
- Carbohydrates: 24g
- Protein: 4g
- Fat: 8g
- Fiber: 5g
- Sugar: 12g

Number of Servings: 6
Cooking Time: 35 minutes

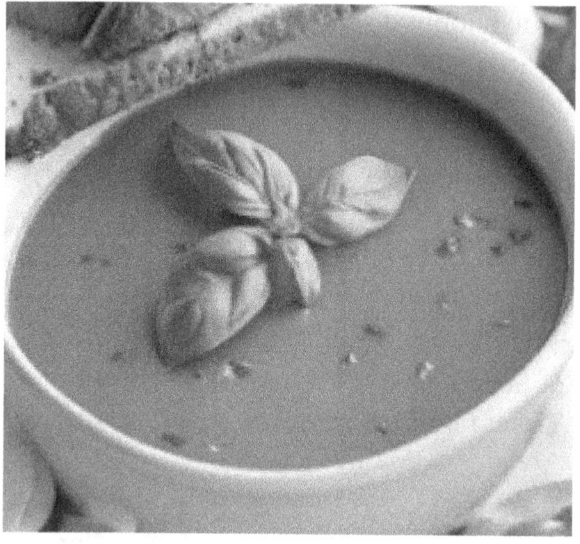

6. Minestrone

Ingredients:
- 2 tablespoons olive oil
- 1 onion, diced
- 2 cloves garlic, minced
- 2 carrots, sliced
- 2 celery stalks, sliced
- 1 zucchini, diced
- 1 can (14.5 ounces) diced tomatoes
- 4 cups low-sodium vegetable broth
- 1 can (15 ounces) kidney beans, drained and rinsed
- 1 cup green beans, trimmed and cut into 1-inch pieces
- 1/2 cup small pasta (such as ditalini or elbow)
- 1 teaspoon dried basil
- 1 teaspoon dried oregano
- 1/4 teaspoon sea salt
- 1/4 teaspoon black pepper
- 1/4 cup fresh parsley, chopped

Instructions:
1. Heat the olive oil in a large pot over medium heat.
2. Add the onion and garlic, and cook for 5-7 minutes until softened.
3. Add the carrots, celery, and zucchini. Cook for another 5 minutes.
4. Stir in the diced tomatoes, vegetable broth, kidney beans, green beans, pasta, dried basil, dried oregano, sea salt, and black pepper. Bring to a boil, then reduce heat and simmer for 15-20 minutes until the vegetables and pasta are tender.
5. Stir in the fresh parsley before serving.
6. Serve warm.

Nutrition Info per Serving:
- Calories: 220
- Carbohydrates: 36g
- Protein: 8g
- Fat: 6g
- Fiber: 8g
- Sugar: 8g

Number of Servings: 6
Cooking Time: 35 minutes

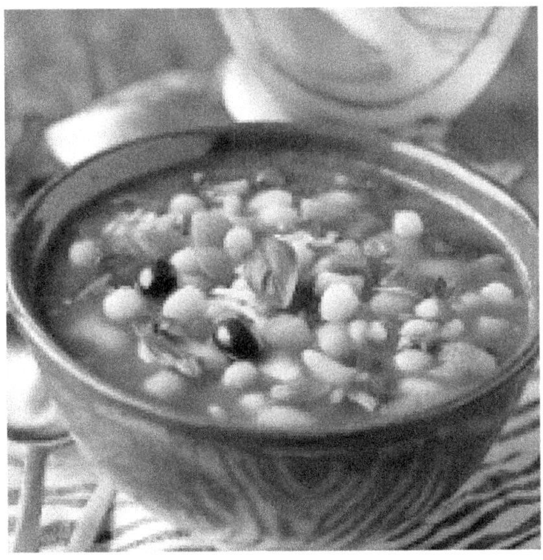

7. Miso Soup

Ingredients:

- 4 cups water
- 1/4 cup miso paste
- 1 package (8 ounces) silken tofu, cubed
- 1 cup sliced shiitake mushrooms
- 1/4 cup chopped green onions
- 1 tablespoon low-sodium soy sauce
- 1 tablespoon wakame seaweed (optional)

Instructions:

1. In a medium pot, bring the water to a simmer.
2. In a small bowl, mix the miso paste with a few tablespoons of hot water until smooth. Add to the pot.
3. Add the cubed tofu, sliced shiitake mushrooms, and soy sauce. Simmer for 5-7 minutes.
4. Stir in the chopped green onions and wakame seaweed (if using).
5. Serve warm.

Nutrition Info per Serving:

- Calories: 80
- Carbohydrates: 6g
- Protein: 6g
- Fat: 4g
- Fiber: 1g
- Sugar: 2g

Number of Servings: 4

Cooking Time: 15 minutes

8. Butternut Squash Soup

Ingredients:

- 2 tablespoons olive oil
- 1 onion, diced
- 3 cloves garlic, minced
- 4 cups butternut squash, peeled and cubed
- 4 cups low-sodium vegetable broth
- 1 teaspoon ground cinnamon
- 1/4 teaspoon ground nutmeg
- 1/4 teaspoon sea salt
- 1/4 teaspoon black pepper
- 1/2 cup coconut milk (optional)

Instructions:

1. Heat the olive oil in a large pot over medium heat.
2. Add the onion and garlic, and cook for 5-7 minutes until softened.
3. Add the butternut squash, vegetable broth, ground cinnamon, ground nutmeg, sea salt, and black pepper. Bring to a boil, then reduce heat and simmer for 20-25 minutes until the squash is tender.
4. Use an immersion blender to puree the soup until smooth (or carefully transfer to a blender in batches).
5. Stir in the coconut milk (if using).
6. Serve warm.

Nutrition Info per Serving:

- Calories: 200
- Carbohydrates: 28g
- Protein: 3g
- Fat: 10g
- Fiber: 6g
- Sugar: 8g

Number of Servings: 6
Cooking Time: 35 minutes

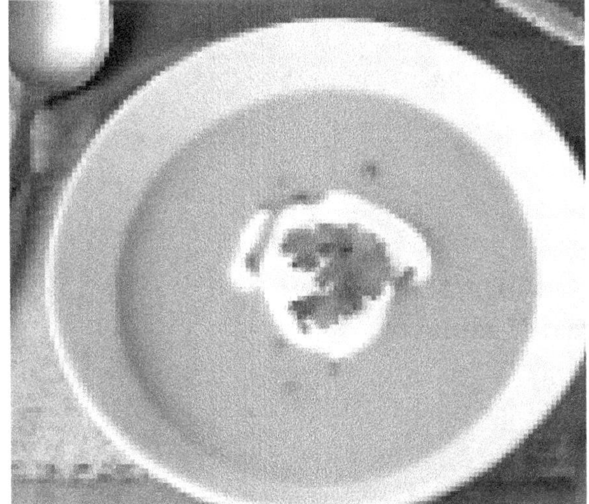

9. Turkey and Rice Soup

Ingredients:

- 1 tablespoon olive oil
- 1 onion, diced
- 2 cloves garlic, minced
- 2 carrots, sliced
- 2 celery stalks, sliced
- 1 pound cooked turkey, shredded
- 6 cups low-sodium chicken broth
- 1/2 cup brown rice
- 1 teaspoon dried thyme
- 1/4 teaspoon sea salt
- 1/4 teaspoon black pepper
- 2 cups chopped spinach

Instructions:

1. Heat the olive oil in a large pot over medium heat.
2. Add the onion and garlic, and cook for 5-7 minutes until softened.
3. Add the carrots and celery, and cook for another 5 minutes.
4. Stir in the shredded turkey, chicken broth, brown rice, dried thyme, sea salt, and black pepper. Bring to a boil, then reduce heat and simmer for 30-35 minutes until the rice is tender.
5. Stir in the chopped spinach and cook for an additional 5 minutes.
6. Serve warm.

Nutrition Info per Serving:

- Calories: 250
- Carbohydrates: 22g
- Protein: 28g
- Fat: 8g
- Fiber: 4g
- Sugar: 4g

Number of Servings: 6
Cooking Time: 45 minutes

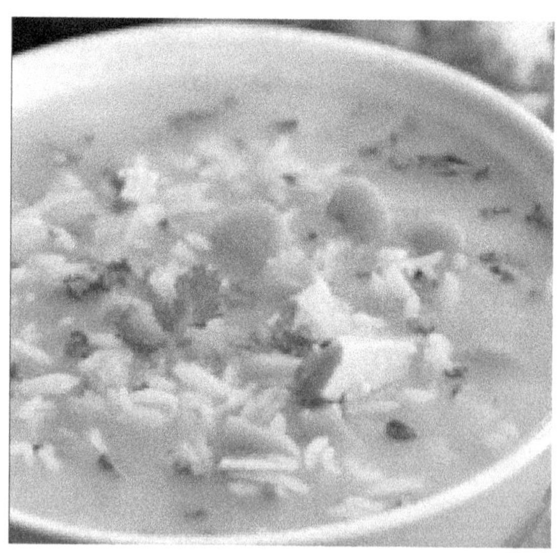

10. Vegetable Beef Stew

Ingredients:

- 1 pound beef stew meat, cut into bite-sized pieces
- 2 tablespoons olive oil
- 1 onion, diced
- 2 cloves garlic, minced
- 2 carrots, sliced
- 2 celery stalks, sliced
- 2 potatoes, peeled and diced
- 1 can (14.5 ounces) diced tomatoes
- 4 cups low-sodium beef broth
- 1 teaspoon dried thyme
- 1/2 teaspoon dried rosemary
- 1/4 teaspoon sea salt
- 1/4 teaspoon black pepper
- 2 cups chopped kale

Instructions:

1. Heat 1 tablespoon of olive oil in a large pot over medium-high heat. Add the beef and cook until browned on all sides. Remove from the pot and set aside.
2. In the same pot, heat the remaining tablespoon of olive oil. Add the onion and garlic, and cook for 5-7 minutes until softened.
3. Add the carrots, celery, and potatoes, and cook for another 5 minutes.
4. Stir in the diced tomatoes, beef broth, dried thyme, dried rosemary, sea salt, and black pepper. Bring to a boil, then reduce heat and simmer for 45 minutes.
5. Return the beef to the pot and simmer for another 15 minutes until the beef is tender and the vegetables are cooked.
6. Stir in the chopped kale and cook for an additional 5 minutes.
7. Serve warm.

Nutrition Info per Serving:

- Calories: 320
- Carbohydrates: 28g
- Protein: 28g
- Fat: 12g
- Fiber: 6g
- Sugar: 6g

Number of Servings: 6

Cooking Time: 1 hour 15 minutes

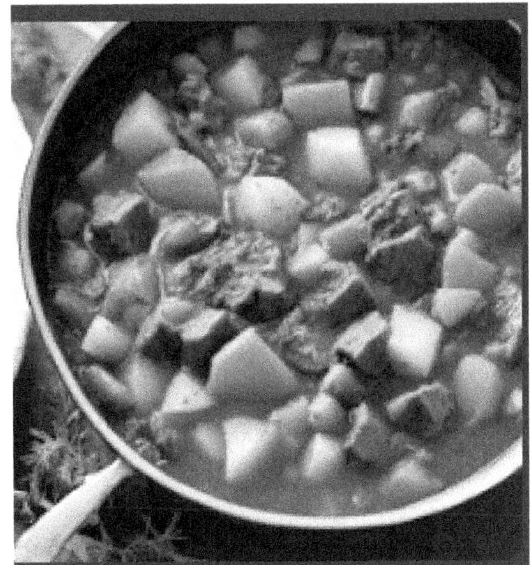

11. Corn Chowder

Ingredients:

- 2 tablespoons olive oil
- 1 onion, diced
- 2 cloves garlic, minced
- 2 cups corn kernels (fresh or frozen)
- 2 potatoes, peeled and diced
- 4 cups low-sodium vegetable broth
- 1 cup unsweetened almond milk
- 1 teaspoon dried thyme
- 1/4 teaspoon sea salt
- 1/4 teaspoon black pepper
- 1/4 cup fresh chives, chopped

Instructions:

1. Heat the olive oil in a large pot over medium heat.
2. Add the onion and garlic, and cook for 5-7 minutes until softened.
3. Add the corn, potatoes, vegetable broth, dried thyme, sea salt, and black pepper. Bring to a boil, then reduce heat and simmer for 20-25 minutes until the potatoes are tender.
4. Use an immersion blender to partially puree the soup, leaving some chunks for texture.
5. Stir in the almond milk and heat through.
6. Garnish with fresh chives before serving.
7. Serve warm.

Nutrition Info per Serving:

- Calories: 180
- Carbohydrates: 32g
- Protein: 4g
- Fat: 6g
- Fiber: 4g
- Sugar: 6g

Number of Servings: 6

Cooking Time: 35 minutes

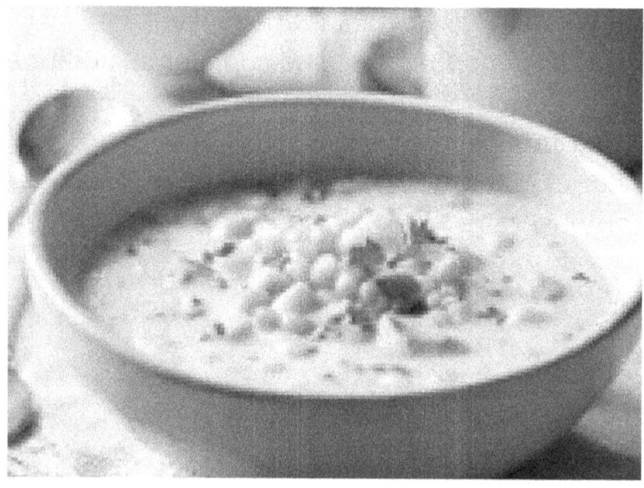

12. French Onion Soup

Ingredients:

- 2 tablespoons olive oil
- 4 large onions, thinly sliced
- 2 cloves garlic, minced
- 1 teaspoon dried thyme
- 1/4 teaspoon sea salt
- 1/4 teaspoon black pepper
- 6 cups low-sodium beef broth
- 1/2 cup dry white wine (optional)
- 1 baguette, sliced and toasted
- 1 cup grated Gruyère cheese

Instructions:

1. Heat the olive oil in a large pot over medium heat.
2. Add the onions and cook, stirring frequently, for 25-30 minutes until caramelized.
3. Add the garlic, dried thyme, sea salt, and black pepper, and cook for another 2 minutes.
4. Stir in the beef broth and white wine (if using). Bring to a boil, then reduce heat and simmer for 20 minutes.
5. Ladle the soup into oven-safe bowls, top with toasted baguette slices, and sprinkle with grated Gruyère cheese.
6. Place the bowls under the broiler for 2-3 minutes until the cheese is melted and bubbly.
7. Serve immediately.

Nutrition Info per Serving:

- Calories: 300
- Carbohydrates: 30g
- Protein: 12g
- Fat: 14g
- Fiber: 4g
- Sugar: 8g

Number of Servings: 6

Cooking Time: 55 minutes

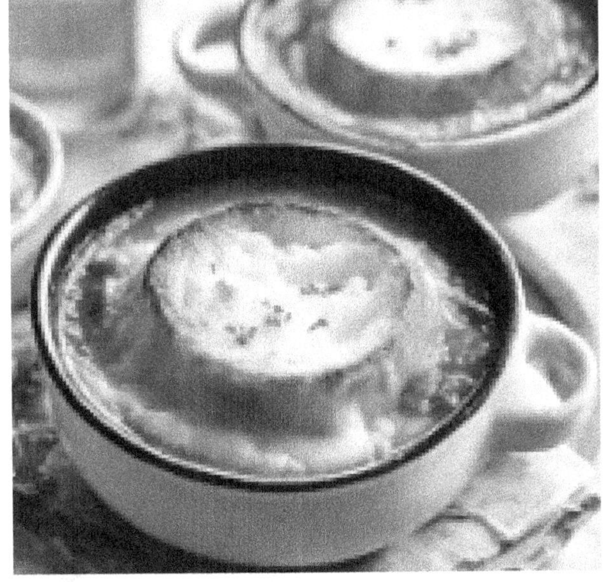

13. White Bean and Kale Soup

Ingredients:

- 2 tablespoons olive oil
- 1 onion, diced
- 2 cloves garlic, minced
- 2 carrots, sliced
- 2 celery stalks, sliced
- 4 cups low-sodium vegetable broth
- 2 cans (15 ounces each) white beans, drained and rinsed
- 1 teaspoon dried thyme
- 1/4 teaspoon sea salt
- 1/4 teaspoon black pepper
- 4 cups chopped kale

Instructions:

1. Heat the olive oil in a large pot over medium heat.
2. Add the onion, garlic, carrots, and celery. Cook for 5-7 minutes until softened.
3. Stir in the vegetable broth, white beans, dried thyme, sea salt, and black pepper. Bring to a boil, then reduce heat and simmer for 20 minutes.
4. Add the chopped kale and cook for another 5 minutes until the kale is tender.
5. Serve warm.

Nutrition Info per Serving:

- Calories: 200
- Carbohydrates: 30g
- Protein: 10g
- Fat: 6g
- Fiber: 8g
- Sugar: 6g

Number of Servings: 6
Cooking Time: 35 minutes

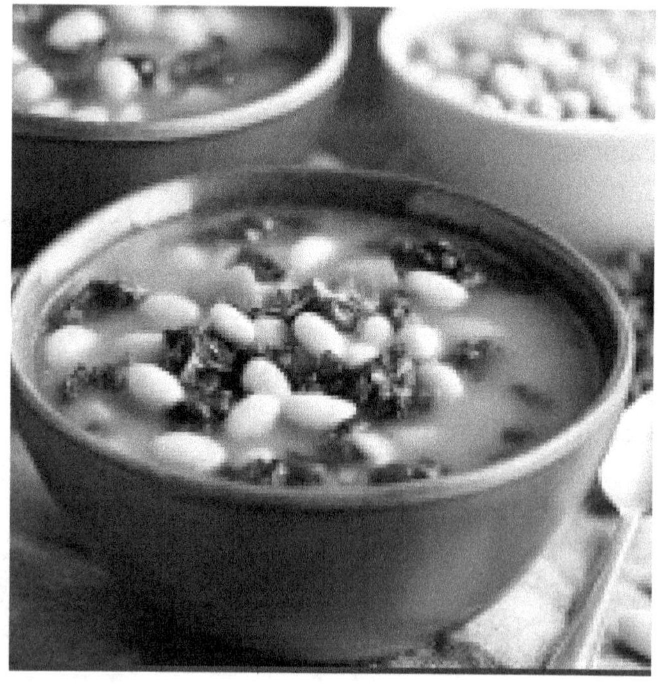

14. Sweet Potato and Black Bean Chili

Ingredients:

- 2 tablespoons olive oil
- 1 onion, diced
- 2 cloves garlic, minced
- 2 large sweet potatoes, peeled and diced
- 1 red bell pepper, diced
- 2 cans (15 ounces each) black beans, drained and rinsed
- 1 can (14.5 ounces) diced tomatoes
- 4 cups low-sodium vegetable broth
- 2 tablespoons chili powder
- 1 teaspoon ground cumin
- 1/4 teaspoon sea salt
- 1/4 teaspoon black pepper
- 1/4 cup fresh cilantro, chopped

Instructions:

1. Heat the olive oil in a large pot over medium heat.
2. Add the onion and garlic, and cook for 5-7 minutes until softened.
3. Add the sweet potatoes and red bell pepper. Cook for another 5 minutes.
4. Stir in the black beans, diced tomatoes, vegetable broth, chili powder, ground cumin, sea salt, and black pepper. Bring to a boil, then reduce heat and simmer for 25-30 minutes until the sweet potatoes are tender.
5. Stir in the fresh cilantro before serving.
6. Serve warm.

Nutrition Info per Serving:

- Calories: 250
- Carbohydrates: 44g
- Protein: 8g
- Fat: 6g
- Fiber: 12g
- Sugar: 10g

Number of Servings: 6

Cooking Time: 40 minutes

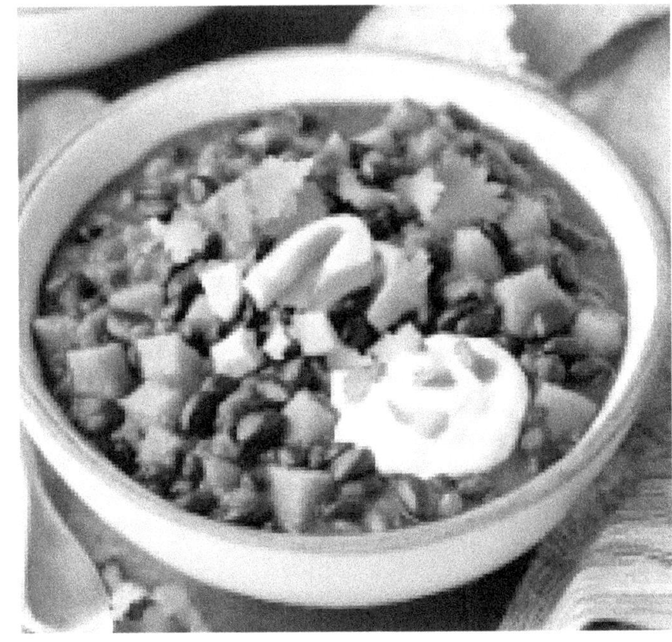

15. Broccoli and Cheddar Soup

Ingredients:

- 2 tablespoons olive oil
- 1 onion, diced
- 2 cloves garlic, minced
- 4 cups broccoli florets
- 4 cups low-sodium vegetable broth
- 1 cup unsweetened almond milk
- 1 teaspoon dried thyme
- 1/4 teaspoon sea salt
- 1/4 teaspoon black pepper
- 1 cup grated sharp cheddar cheese

Instructions:

1. Heat the olive oil in a large pot over medium heat.
2. Add the onion and garlic, and cook for 5-7 minutes until softened.
3. Add the broccoli, vegetable broth, dried thyme, sea salt, and black pepper. Bring to a boil, then reduce heat and simmer for 15-20 minutes until the broccoli is tender.
4. Use an immersion blender to partially puree the soup, leaving some chunks for texture.
5. Stir in the almond milk and grated cheddar cheese. Cook until the cheese is melted and the soup is heated through.
6. Serve warm.

Nutrition Info per Serving:

- Calories: 220
- Carbohydrates: 14g
- Protein: 8g
- Fat: 16g
- Fiber: 4g
- Sugar: 4g

Number of Servings: 6

Cooking Time: 30 minutes

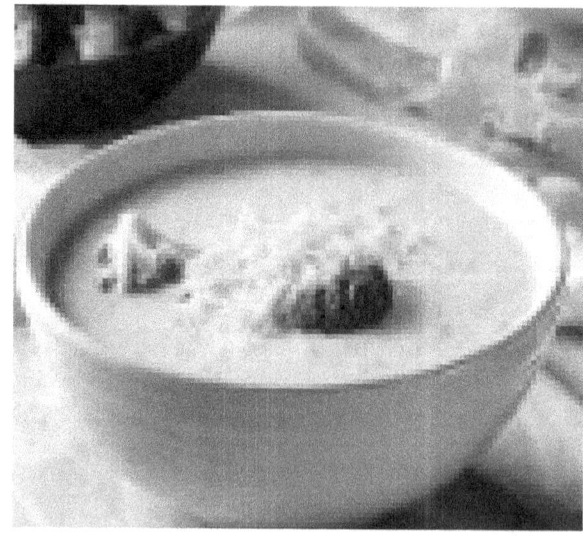

16. Pea and Ham Soup

Ingredients:

- 1 tablespoon olive oil
- 1 onion, diced
- 2 cloves garlic, minced
- 2 cups dried split peas, rinsed
- 6 cups low-sodium chicken broth
- 1 cup diced ham
- 2 carrots, sliced
- 2 celery stalks, sliced
- 1 teaspoon dried thyme
- 1/4 teaspoon sea salt
- 1/4 teaspoon black pepper

Instructions:

1. Heat the olive oil in a large pot over medium heat.
2. Add the onion and garlic, and cook for 5-7 minutes until softened.
3. Add the split peas, chicken broth, diced ham, carrots, celery, dried thyme, sea salt, and black pepper. Bring to a boil, then reduce heat and simmer for 1 hour until the peas are tender and the soup has thickened.
4. Serve warm.

Nutrition Info per Serving:

- Calories: 280
- Carbohydrates: 36g
- Protein: 18g
- Fat: 8g
- Fiber: 12g
- Sugar: 6g

Number of Servings: 6
Cooking Time: 1 hour 15 minutes

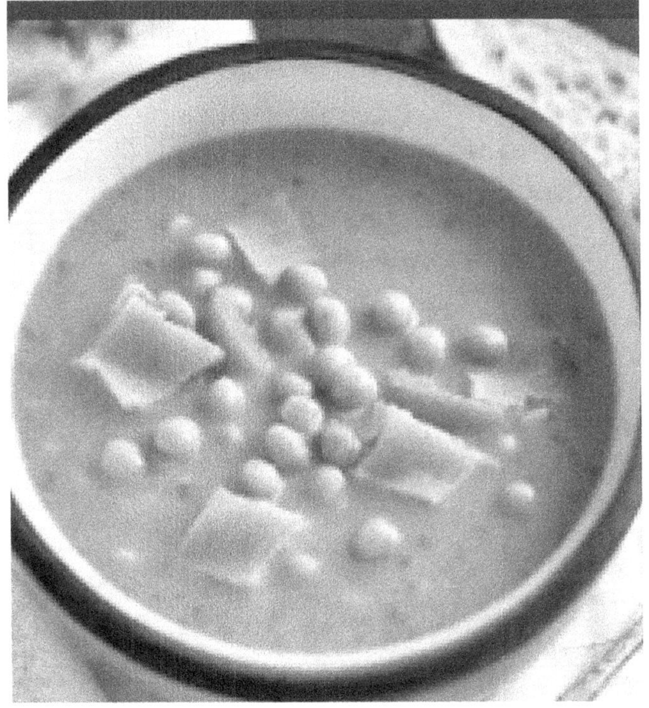

17. Clam Chowder
Ingredients:

- 2 tablespoons olive oil
- 1 onion, diced
- 2 cloves garlic, minced
- 2 celery stalks, sliced
- 2 potatoes, peeled and diced
- 2 cups clams, chopped (fresh or canned)
- 4 cups low-sodium vegetable broth
- 1 cup unsweetened almond milk
- 1 teaspoon dried thyme
- 1/4 teaspoon sea salt
- 1/4 teaspoon black pepper
- 1 bay leaf
- 1/4 cup fresh parsley, chopped

Instructions:

1. Heat the olive oil in a large pot over medium heat.
2. Add the onion, garlic, and celery. Cook for 5-7 minutes until softened.
3. Add the potatoes, clams, vegetable broth, dried thyme, sea salt, black pepper, and bay leaf. Bring to a boil, then reduce heat and simmer for 20-25 minutes until the potatoes are tender.
4. Stir in the almond milk and cook for an additional 5 minutes.
5. Remove the bay leaf before serving.
6. Garnish with fresh parsley.
7. Serve warm.

Nutrition Info per Serving:

- Calories: 200
- Carbohydrates: 20g
- Protein: 12g
- Fat: 8g
- Fiber: 3g
- Sugar: 4g

Number of Servings: 6
Cooking Time: 35 minutes

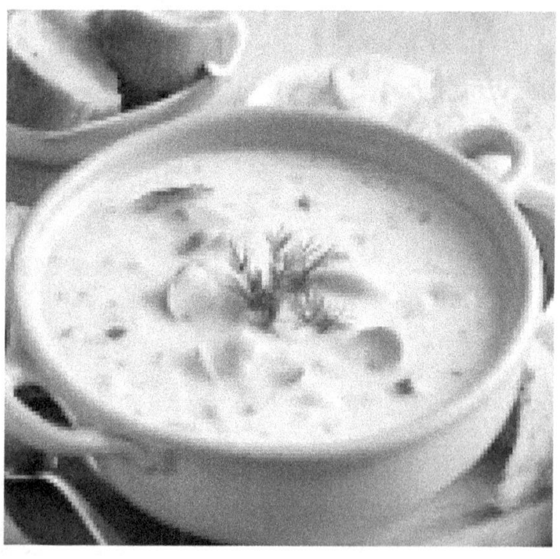

18. Borscht

Ingredients:

- 2 tablespoons olive oil
- 1 onion, diced
- 2 cloves garlic, minced
- 3 beets, peeled and grated
- 2 carrots, peeled and grated
- 1 potato, peeled and diced
- 4 cups low-sodium vegetable broth
- 1 can (14.5 ounces) diced tomatoes
- 1 teaspoon dried dill
- 1/4 teaspoon sea salt
- 1/4 teaspoon black pepper
- 2 tablespoons apple cider vinegar
- 1/4 cup fresh dill, chopped (for garnish)
- 1/4 cup sour cream (optional, for garnish)

Instructions:

1. Heat the olive oil in a large pot over medium heat.
2. Add the onion and garlic. Cook for 5-7 minutes until softened.
3. Add the grated beets, grated carrots, and diced potato. Cook for another 5 minutes.
4. Stir in the vegetable broth, diced tomatoes, dried dill, sea salt, and black pepper. Bring to a boil, then reduce heat and simmer for 30-35 minutes until the vegetables are tender.
5. Stir in the apple cider vinegar.
6. Garnish with fresh dill and a dollop of sour cream (if using).
7. Serve warm.

Nutrition Info per Serving:

- Calories: 150
- Carbohydrates: 24g
- Protein: 3g
- Fat: 6g
- Fiber: 5g
- Sugar: 12g

Number of Servings: 6

Cooking Time: 45 minutes

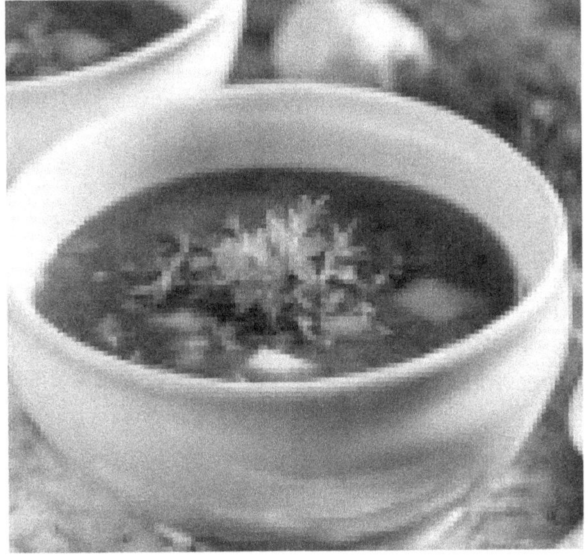

19. Italian Wedding Soup
Ingredients:
- 1 tablespoon olive oil
- 1 onion, diced
- 2 cloves garlic, minced
- 2 carrots, sliced
- 2 celery stalks, sliced
- 1 pound ground turkey
- 1/4 cup whole wheat breadcrumbs
- 1 egg, beaten
- 1 teaspoon dried oregano
- 1/4 teaspoon sea salt
- 1/4 teaspoon black pepper
- 6 cups low-sodium chicken broth
- 1/2 cup small pasta (such as acini di pepe or orzo)
- 4 cups spinach, chopped
- 1/4 cup grated Parmesan cheese (optional)

Instructions:
1. In a bowl, mix together the ground turkey, whole wheat breadcrumbs, beaten egg, dried oregano, sea salt, and black pepper. Form into small meatballs.
2. Heat the olive oil in a large pot over medium heat. Add the onion and garlic. Cook for 5-7 minutes until softened.
3. Add the carrots and celery. Cook for another 5 minutes.
4. Stir in the chicken broth and bring to a boil. Add the meatballs and pasta. Reduce heat and simmer for 10-12 minutes until the meatballs are cooked through and the pasta is tender.
5. Stir in the chopped spinach and cook for an additional 2-3 minutes.
6. Serve warm, garnished with grated Parmesan cheese if desired.

Nutrition Info per Serving:
- Calories: 250
- Carbohydrates: 20g
- Protein: 24g
- Fat: 10g
- Fiber: 3g
- Sugar: 4g

Number of Servings: 6
Cooking Time: 30 minutes

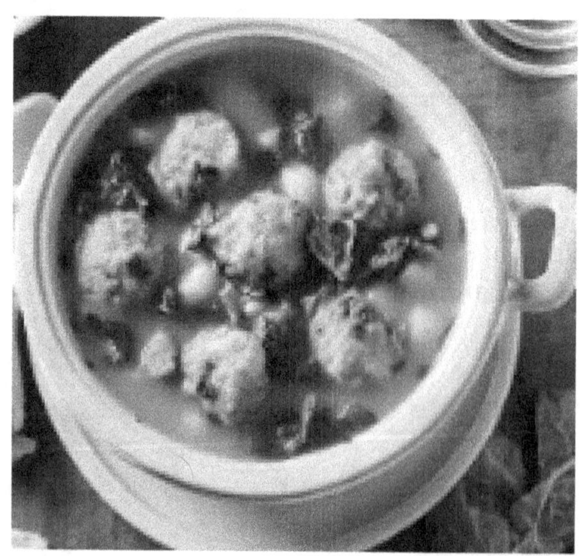

20. Mulligatawny Soup

Ingredients:

- 2 tablespoons olive oil
- 1 onion, diced
- 2 cloves garlic, minced
- 1 tablespoon fresh ginger, grated
- 2 carrots, sliced
- 1 apple, peeled and diced
- 1 pound boneless, skinless chicken breasts, cut into bite-sized pieces
- 1 tablespoon curry powder
- 1/2 teaspoon ground cumin
- 4 cups low-sodium chicken broth
- 1 cup unsweetened coconut milk
- 1/4 cup basmati rice
- 1/4 teaspoon sea salt
- 1/4 teaspoon black pepper
- 1/4 cup fresh cilantro, chopped

Instructions:

1. Heat the olive oil in a large pot over medium heat. Add the onion, garlic, and fresh ginger. Cook for 5-7 minutes until softened.
2. Add the carrots, apple, and chicken pieces. Cook for another 5 minutes.
3. Stir in the curry powder and ground cumin. Cook for 1 minute until fragrant.
4. Add the chicken broth, coconut milk, basmati rice, sea salt, and black pepper. Bring to a boil, then reduce heat and simmer for 20-25 minutes until the chicken is cooked through and the rice is tender.
5. Garnish with fresh cilantro before serving.
6. Serve warm.

Nutrition Info per Serving:

- Calories: 300
- Carbohydrates: 22g
- Protein: 28g
- Fat: 12g
- Fiber: 3g
- Sugar: 6g

Number of Servings: 6
Cooking Time: 35 minutes

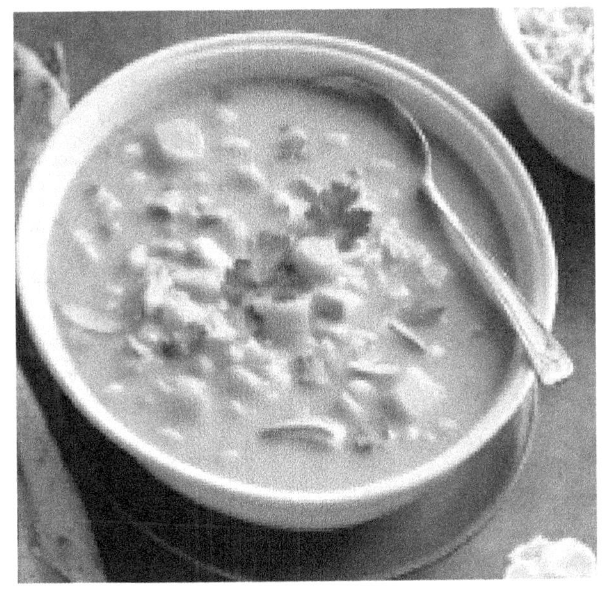

21. Mushroom Barley Soup

Ingredients:

- 2 tablespoons olive oil
- 1 onion, diced
- 2 cloves garlic, minced
- 2 cups mushrooms, sliced
- 2 carrots, sliced
- 2 celery stalks, sliced
- 1 cup pearl barley
- 6 cups low-sodium vegetable broth
- 1 teaspoon dried thyme
- 1/4 teaspoon sea salt
- 1/4 teaspoon black pepper
- 1/4 cup fresh parsley, chopped

Instructions:

1. Heat the olive oil in a large pot over medium heat. Add the onion and garlic. Cook for 5-7 minutes until softened.
2. Add the mushrooms, carrots, and celery. Cook for another 5 minutes.
3. Stir in the pearl barley, vegetable broth, dried thyme, sea salt, and black pepper. Bring to a boil, then reduce heat and simmer for 45 minutes until the barley is tender.
4. Garnish with fresh parsley before serving.
5. Serve warm.

Nutrition Info per Serving:

- Calories: 220
- Carbohydrates: 38g
- Protein: 6g
- Fat: 7g
- Fiber: 8g
- Sugar: 6g

Number of Servings: 6
Cooking Time: 55 minutes

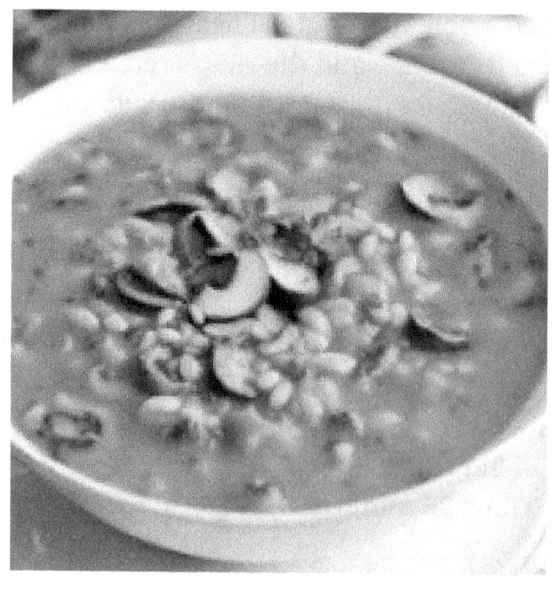

22. Zucchini Soup

Ingredients:

- 2 tablespoons olive oil
- 1 onion, diced
- 2 cloves garlic, minced
- 4 medium zucchinis, sliced
- 4 cups low-sodium vegetable broth
- 1 teaspoon dried thyme
- 1/4 teaspoon sea salt
- 1/4 teaspoon black pepper
- 1/4 cup fresh basil, chopped
- 1/2 cup unsweetened almond milk (optional)

Instructions:

1. Heat the olive oil in a large pot over medium heat.
2. Add the onion and garlic, and cook for 5-7 minutes until softened.
3. Add the sliced zucchinis, vegetable broth, dried thyme, sea salt, and black pepper. Bring to a boil, then reduce heat and simmer for 20-25 minutes until the zucchinis are tender.
4. Use an immersion blender to puree the soup until smooth (or carefully transfer to a blender in batches).
5. Stir in the fresh basil and almond milk (if using).
6. Serve warm.

Nutrition Info per Serving:

- Calories: 110
- Carbohydrates: 14g
- Protein: 3g
- Fat: 6g
- Fiber: 3g
- Sugar: 6g

Number of Servings: 6

Cooking Time: 30 minutes

23. Beet and Cabbage Stew
Ingredients:
- 2 tablespoons olive oil
- 1 onion, diced
- 2 cloves garlic, minced
- 3 medium beets, peeled and diced
- 2 cups cabbage, shredded
- 2 carrots, sliced
- 4 cups low-sodium vegetable broth
- 1 can (14.5 ounces) diced tomatoes
- 1 teaspoon dried dill
- 1/4 teaspoon sea salt
- 1/4 teaspoon black pepper
- 2 tablespoons apple cider vinegar
- 1/4 cup fresh dill, chopped (for garnish)

Instructions:
1. Heat the olive oil in a large pot over medium heat.
2. Add the onion and garlic, and cook for 5-7 minutes until softened.
3. Add the beets, cabbage, and carrots. Cook for another 5 minutes.
4. Stir in the vegetable broth, diced tomatoes, dried dill, sea salt, and black pepper. Bring to a boil, then reduce heat and simmer for 30-35 minutes until the vegetables are tender.
5. Stir in the apple cider vinegar.
6. Garnish with fresh dill before serving.
7. Serve warm.

Nutrition Info per Serving:
- Calories: 140
- Carbohydrates: 23g
- Protein: 3g
- Fat: 5g
- Fiber: 6g
- Sugar: 12g

Number of Servings: 6
Cooking Time: 45 minutes

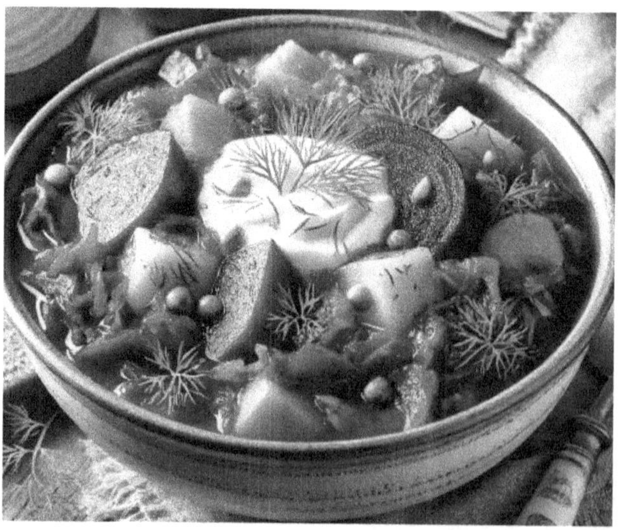

24. Black Bean Soup

Ingredients:

- 2 tablespoons olive oil
- 1 onion, diced
- 2 cloves garlic, minced
- 1 red bell pepper, diced
- 1 green bell pepper, diced
- 2 cans (15 ounces each) black beans, drained and rinsed
- 4 cups low-sodium vegetable broth
- 1 teaspoon ground cumin
- 1 teaspoon chili powder
- 1/4 teaspoon sea salt
- 1/4 teaspoon black pepper
- 1 tablespoon lime juice
- 1/4 cup fresh cilantro, chopped

Instructions:

1. Heat the olive oil in a large pot over medium heat.
2. Add the onion and garlic, and cook for 5-7 minutes until softened.
3. Add the red and green bell peppers, and cook for another 5 minutes.
4. Stir in the black beans, vegetable broth, ground cumin, chili powder, sea salt, and black pepper. Bring to a boil, then reduce heat and simmer for 20-25 minutes.
5. Use an immersion blender to partially puree the soup, leaving some chunks for texture.
6. Stir in the lime juice.
7. Garnish with fresh cilantro before serving.
8. Serve warm.

Nutrition Info per Serving:

- Calories: 210
- Carbohydrates: 34g
- Protein: 9g
- Fat: 7g
- Fiber: 12g
- Sugar: 4g

Number of Servings: 6
Cooking Time: 35 minutes

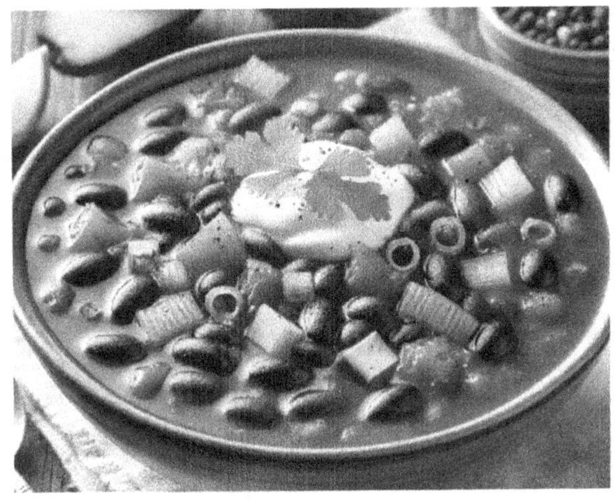

25. Italian Sausage Soup

Ingredients:

- 1 pound Italian turkey sausage, casings removed
- 2 tablespoons olive oil
- 1 onion, diced
- 2 cloves garlic, minced
- 2 carrots, sliced
- 2 celery stalks, sliced
- 4 cups low-sodium chicken broth
- 1 can (14.5 ounces) diced tomatoes
- 1 teaspoon dried basil
- 1 teaspoon dried oregano
- 1/4 teaspoon sea salt
- 1/4 teaspoon black pepper
- 1 cup small pasta (such as ditalini or elbow)
- 4 cups spinach, chopped

Instructions:

1. Heat the olive oil in a large pot over medium heat.
2. Add the Italian turkey sausage and cook, breaking it up with a spoon, until browned.
3. Add the onion and garlic, and cook for 5-7 minutes until softened.
4. Stir in the carrots and celery, and cook for another 5 minutes.
5. Add the chicken broth, diced tomatoes, dried basil, dried oregano, sea salt, and black pepper. Bring to a boil, then reduce heat and simmer for 15-20 minutes.
6. Stir in the pasta and cook for another 10 minutes until the pasta is tender.
7. Add the chopped spinach and cook for an additional 2-3 minutes.
8. Serve warm.

Nutrition Info per Serving:

- Calories: 290
- Carbohydrates: 25g
- Protein: 20g
- Fat: 12g
- Fiber: 4g
- Sugar: 6g

Number of Servings: 6
Cooking Time: 40 minutes

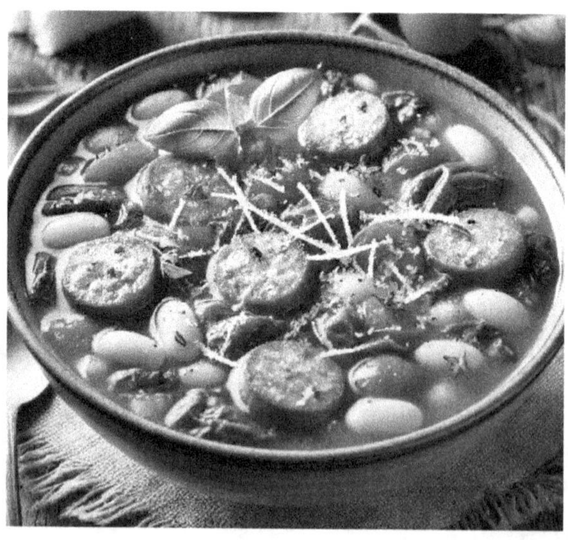

10-WEEK MEAL PLAN

Week 1
Monday
- Breakfast: Mixed Vegetable Juice
- Lunch: Grilled Chicken Salad
- Dinner: Lentil Soup

Tuesday
- Breakfast: Tomato and Basil Bruschetta
- Lunch: Baked Cod with Olive Tapenade
- Dinner: Chicken Ratatouille

Wednesday
- Breakfast: Savory Millet Porridge
- Lunch: Mediterranean Stuffed Chicken
- Dinner: Carrot and Ginger Soup

Thursday
- Breakfast: Papaya and Lime Salad
- Lunch: Turkey and Sweet Potato Skillet
- Dinner: Split Pea Soup

Friday
- Breakfast: Green Tea Smoothie
- Lunch: Grilled Salmon with Dill
- Dinner: Beef Barley Soup

Saturday
- Breakfast: Raspberry Ricotta Toast
- Lunch: Chicken Bruschetta
- Dinner: Zucchini Soup

Sunday
- Breakfast: Almond and Date Porridge
- Lunch: Shrimp Stir-Fry with Vegetables
- Dinner: Butternut Squash Soup

Week 2
Monday
- Breakfast: Overnight Chia and Oats
- Lunch: Mackerel Salad
- Dinner: Black Bean Soup

Tuesday
- Breakfast: Salmon and Cream Cheese Bagel
- Lunch: Fish Tacos with Cabbage Slaw
- Dinner: French Onion Soup

Wednesday
- Breakfast: Zucchini Bread
- Lunch: Tilapia in Parchment
- Dinner: White Bean and Kale Soup

Thursday
- Breakfast: Beetroot and Berry Smoothie
- Lunch: Moroccan Chicken Tagine
- Dinner: Sweet Potato and Black Bean Chili

Friday
- Breakfast: Blueberry and Lemon Muffins
- Lunch: Grilled Tuna Steak
- Dinner: Broccoli and Cheddar Soup

Saturday
- Breakfast: Bircher Muesli
- Lunch: Turkey Meatballs in Tomato Sauce
- Dinner: Pea and Ham Soup

Sunday
- Breakfast: Pear and Walnut Baked Oatmeal
- Lunch: Seafood Paella
- Dinner: Borscht

Week 3

Monday
- Breakfast: Mushroom and Zucchini Saute
- Lunch: Chicken Cacciatore
- Dinner: Italian Wedding Soup

Tuesday
- Breakfast: Pumpkin Smoothie
- Lunch: Turkey Stuffed Peppers
- Dinner: Mulligatawny Soup

Wednesday
- Breakfast: Apple-Cinnamon Steel-Cut Oats
- Lunch: Turkey and Rice Soup
- Dinner: Corn Chowder

Thursday
- Breakfast: Kale and Sweet Onion Frittata
- Lunch: Balsamic Glazed Chicken
- Dinner: Clam Chowder

Friday
- Breakfast: Rice Cake with Almond Butter
- Lunch: Italian Sausage Soup
- Dinner: Chicken Curry with Coconut Milk

Saturday
- Breakfast: Buckwheat Pancakes
- Lunch: Fish Stew with Vegetables
- Dinner: Beet and Cabbage Stew

Sunday
- Breakfast: Muesli and Skim Milk
- Lunch: Grilled Mahi Mahi with Mango Salsa
- Dinner: Chicken Paillard

Week 4

Monday
- Breakfast: Yogurt with Mixed Nuts and Berries
- Lunch: Pesto Halibut
- Dinner: Mushroom Barley Soup

Tuesday
- Breakfast: Quinoa Porridge
- Lunch: Scallop Pasta with Asparagus
- Dinner: Barbecue Chicken Breast

Wednesday
- Breakfast: Sweet Potato Hash
- Lunch: Baked Snapper with Citrus
- Dinner: Chicken Piccata

Thursday
- Breakfast: Banana Pancakes
- Lunch: Turkey Soup with Kale
- Dinner: Chicken Lettuce Wraps

Friday
- Breakfast: Mixed Vegetable Juice
- Lunch: Chicken Bruschetta
- Dinner: Black Bean Soup

Saturday
- Breakfast: Tomato and Basil Bruschetta
- Lunch: Chicken Ratatouille
- Dinner: Zucchini Soup

Sunday
- Breakfast: Savory Millet Porridge
- Lunch: Grilled Tuna Steak
- Dinner: Butternut Squash Soup

Week 5

Monday
- Breakfast: Papaya and Lime Salad
- Lunch: Mackerel Salad
- Dinner: Pea and Ham Soup

Tuesday
- Breakfast: Green Tea Smoothie
- Lunch: Chicken Cacciatore
- Dinner: Sweet Potato and Black Bean Chili

Wednesday
- Breakfast: Raspberry Ricotta Toast
- Lunch: Italian Sausage Soup
- Dinner: Corn Chowder

Thursday
- Breakfast: Almond and Date Porridge
- Lunch: Moroccan Chicken Tagine
- Dinner: Broccoli and Cheddar Soup

Friday
- Breakfast: Overnight Chia and Oats
- Lunch: Fish Tacos with Cabbage Slaw
- Dinner: Mulligatawny Soup

Saturday
- Breakfast: Salmon and Cream Cheese Bagel
- Lunch: Grilled Salmon with Dill
- Dinner: Chicken Curry with Coconut Milk

Sunday
- Breakfast: Zucchini Bread
- Lunch: Turkey Meatballs in Tomato Sauce
- Dinner: Mushroom Barley Soup

Week 6

Monday
- Breakfast: Beetroot and Berry Smoothie
- Lunch: Turkey Meatballs in Tomato Sauce
- Dinner: Sweet Potato and Black Bean Chili

Tuesday
- Breakfast: Blueberry and Lemon Muffins
- Lunch: Fish Stew with Vegetables
- Dinner: Broccoli and Cheddar Soup

Wednesday
- Breakfast: Bircher Muesli
- Lunch: Clam Chowder
- Dinner: Chicken Ratatouille

Thursday
- Breakfast: Pear and Walnut Baked Oatmeal
- Lunch: Baked Snapper with Citrus
- Dinner: Black Bean Soup

Friday
- Breakfast: Mushroom and Zucchini Saute
- Lunch: Italian Sausage Soup
- Dinner: Butternut Squash Soup

Saturday
- Breakfast: Pumpkin Smoothie
- Lunch: Pesto Halibut
- Dinner: Mushroom Barley Soup

Sunday
- Breakfast: Apple-Cinnamon Steel-Cut Oats
- Lunch: Chicken Bruschetta
- Dinner: Mulligatawny Soup

Week 7

Monday
- Breakfast: Kale and Sweet Onion Frittata
- Lunch: Grilled Tuna Steak
- Dinner: Chicken Piccata

Tuesday
- Breakfast: Rice Cake with Almond Butter
- Lunch: Scallop Pasta with Asparagus
- Dinner: Corn Chowder

Wednesday
- Breakfast: Buckwheat Pancakes
- Lunch: Moroccan Chicken Tagine
- Dinner: Pea and Ham Soup

Thursday
- Breakfast: Muesli and Skim Milk
- Lunch: Grilled Mahi Mahi with Mango Salsa
- Dinner: Chicken Paillard

Friday
- Breakfast: Yogurt with Mixed Nuts and Berries
- Lunch: Seafood Paella
- Dinner: French Onion Soup

Saturday

- Breakfast: Quinoa Porridge
- Lunch: Barbecue Chicken Breast
- Dinner: Italian Wedding Soup

Sunday

- Breakfast: Sweet Potato Hash
- Lunch: Shrimp Stir-Fry with Vegetables
- Dinner: Lentil Soup

Week 8

Monday

- Breakfast: Banana Pancakes
- Lunch: Pesto Halibut
- Dinner: Tomato Basil Soup

Tuesday

- Breakfast: Mixed Vegetable Juice
- Lunch: Fish Tacos with Cabbage Slaw
- Dinner: Beef Barley Soup

Wednesday

- Breakfast: Tomato and Basil Bruschetta
- Lunch: Clam Chowder
- Dinner: White Bean and Kale Soup

Thursday

- Breakfast: Savory Millet Porridge
- Lunch: Chicken Ratatouille
- Dinner: Borscht

Friday

- Breakfast: Papaya and Lime Salad
- Lunch: Scallop Pasta with Asparagus
- Dinner: Sweet Potato and Black Bean Chili

Saturday

- Breakfast: Green Tea Smoothie
- Lunch: Italian Sausage Soup
- Dinner: Mulligatawny Soup

Sunday

- Breakfast: Raspberry Ricotta Toast
- Lunch: Grilled Tuna Steak
- Dinner: Mushroom Barley Soup

Week 9

Monday
- Breakfast: Almond and Date Porridge
- Lunch: Mediterranean Stuffed Chicken
- Dinner: Black Bean Soup

Tuesday
- Breakfast: Overnight Chia and Oats
- Lunch: Grilled Salmon with Dill
- Dinner: Broccoli and Cheddar Soup

Wednesday
- Breakfast: Salmon and Cream Cheese Bagel
- Lunch: Fish Stew with Vegetables
- Dinner: Carrot and Ginger Soup

Thursday
- Breakfast: Zucchini Bread
- Lunch: Chicken Bruschetta
- Dinner: Tomato Basil Soup

Friday
- Breakfast: Beetroot and Berry Smoothie
- Lunch: Turkey and Sweet Potato Skillet
- Dinner: Split Pea Soup

Saturday
- Breakfast: Blueberry and Lemon Muffins
- Lunch: Shrimp Stir-Fry with Vegetables
- Dinner: Butternut Squash Soup

Sunday
- Breakfast: Bircher Muesli
- Lunch: Chicken Curry with Coconut Milk
- Dinner: Borscht

Week 10

Monday
- Breakfast: Pear and Walnut Baked Oatmeal
- Lunch: Tilapia in Parchment
- Dinner: Lentil Soup

Tuesday
- Breakfast: Mushroom and Zucchini Saute
- Lunch: Turkey Meatballs in Tomato Sauce
- Dinner: Sweet Potato and Black Bean Chili

Wednesday

- Breakfast: Pumpkin Smoothie
- Lunch: Grilled Mahi Mahi with Mango Salsa
- Dinner: Pea and Ham Soup

Thursday

- Breakfast: Apple-Cinnamon Steel-Cut Oats
- Lunch: Grilled Tuna Steak
- Dinner: White Bean and Kale Soup

Friday

- Breakfast: Kale and Sweet Onion Frittata
- Lunch: Pesto Halibut
- Dinner: French Onion Soup

Saturday

- Breakfast: Rice Cake with Almond Butter
- Lunch: Chicken Bruschetta
- Dinner: Italian Wedding Soup

Sunday

- Breakfast: Buckwheat Pancakes
- Lunch: Moroccan Chicken Tagine
- Dinner: Black Bean Soup

WEEKLY MEAL PLANNER + WORKBOOK

	BREAKFAST	LUNCH	DINNER	SNACKS
MONDAY				
TUESDAY				
WEDNESDAY				
THURSDAY				
FRIDAY				
SATURDAY				
SUNDAY				

Describe your current daily eating habits. What types of foods do you typically eat for breakfast, lunch, and dinner?

WEEKLY MEAL PLANNER + WORKBOOK

	BREAKFAST	LUNCH	DINNER	SNACKS
MONDAY				
TUESDAY				
WEDNESDAY				
THURSDAY				
FRIDAY				
SATURDAY				
SUNDAY				

How much water do you drink each day? Can you identify ways to increase your water intake if needed?

WEEKLY MEAL PLANNER + WORKBOOK

	BREAKFAST	LUNCH	DINNER	SNACKS
MONDAY				
TUESDAY				
WEDNESDAY				
THURSDAY				
FRIDAY				
SATURDAY				
SUNDAY				

Do you currently prepare your meals at home or rely on pre-prepared meals? What challenges do you face with meal preparation?

....

....

....

....

....

....

WEEKLY MEAL PLANNER + WORKBOOK

	BREAKFAST	LUNCH	DINNER	SNACKS
MONDAY				
TUESDAY				
WEDNESDAY				
THURSDAY				
FRIDAY				
SATURDAY				
SUNDAY				

List your favorite foods. Are these foods part of the recommended Parkinson's disease diet?

WEEKLY MEAL PLANNER + WORKBOOK

	BREAKFAST	LUNCH	DINNER	SNACKS
MONDAY				
TUESDAY				
WEDNESDAY				
THURSDAY				
FRIDAY				
SATURDAY				
SUNDAY				

Describe your grocery shopping habits. Do you read nutrition labels? How do you plan your grocery list?

WEEKLY MEAL PLANNER + WORKBOOK

	BREAKFAST	LUNCH	DINNER	SNACKS
MONDAY				
TUESDAY				
WEDNESDAY				
THURSDAY				
FRIDAY				
SATURDAY				
SUNDAY				

Rate your confidence in your cooking skills. What new recipes or cooking techniques would you like to learn?

WEEKLY MEAL PLANNER + WORKBOOK

	BREAKFAST	LUNCH	DINNER	SNACKS
MONDAY				
TUESDAY				
WEDNESDAY				
THURSDAY				
FRIDAY				
SATURDAY				
SUNDAY				

How often do you eat out at restaurants? What strategies can you use to make healthier choices when dining out?

WEEKLY MEAL PLANNER + WORKBOOK

	BREAKFAST	LUNCH	DINNER	SNACKS
MONDAY				
TUESDAY				
WEDNESDAY				
THURSDAY				
FRIDAY				
SATURDAY				
SUNDAY				

How do you feel after eating different types of meals? Are there specific foods that make you feel better or worse?

....

....

....

....

....

WEEKLY MEAL PLANNER + WORKBOOK

	BREAKFAST	LUNCH	DINNER	SNACKS
MONDAY				
TUESDAY				
WEDNESDAY				
THURSDAY				
FRIDAY				
SATURDAY				
SUNDAY				

After following the Parkinson's disease diet for one month, reflect on your progress. What positive changes have you noticed? What challenges have you faced, and how can you address them moving forward?

....

....

....

....

....

....

Scan the QR code below to get a surprise bonus!

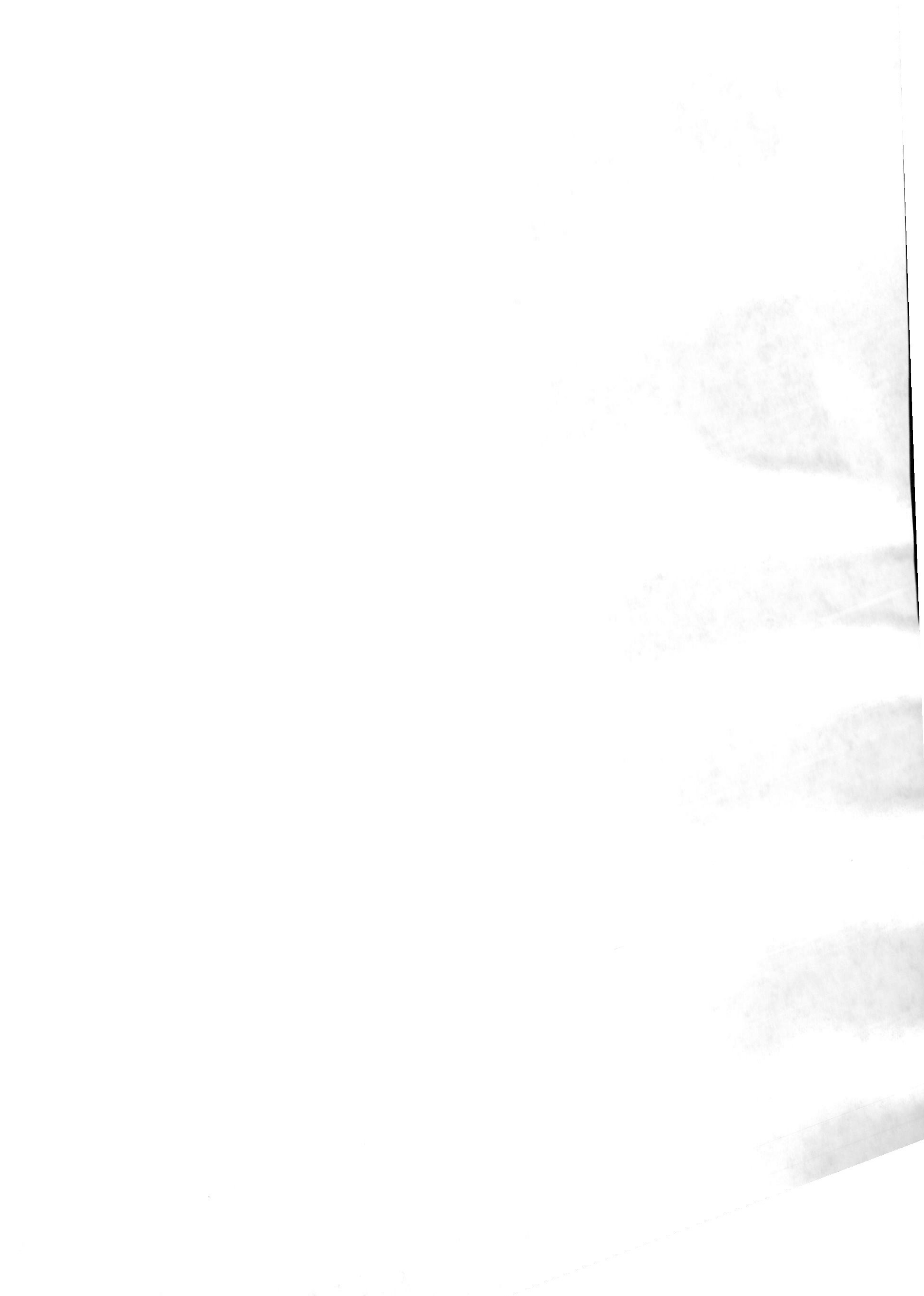